Michael D. Huggins

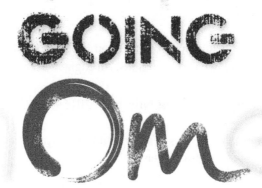

GOING
hOme

A CEO's Journey from Prison
Facility to Spiritual Tranquility

Hawkeye Publishers

Library of Congress Control Number: 2016959873

Author Photograph by Chris Leaman Photography
Cover Design by Kate Hunsinger

For more information, address Hawkeye Publishers
P.O. Box 3098, Camarillo, CA 93011.

Paperback: 978-1946005090
Hardcover: 978-1946005038
Ebook: 978-1946005045

HAWKEYEPUBLISHERS.COM

This book is dedicated to my brother, Bob.
I wish you were still here.

Keep in mind...

This is my recollection of events that changed my life.

Others involved in these events may have different memories of them, but this is how I saw my journey.

The names of most of the characters have been changed to protect their privacy.

Mike Huggins

Table of Contents

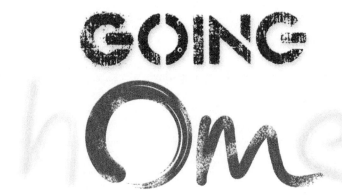

Foreword by Gabriel

(Serving a life sentence at a maximum-security Pennsylvania State Correctional Facility, Fall 2016)

Inspiring Michael D. Huggins takes us on a journey through the levels of human consciousness and devotion that can only be realized during some of the most trying times in our lives.

Having ascended the metaphorical ladder that society correlates with success, Mr. Huggins, or "Hugs," as I've come to know him, provides a unique perspective of life as a corporate CEO and respected member of the community.

But when his life suddenly comes crashing down, Huggins is stripped of his titles and luxuries. He finds himself placed in federal prison for a misdemeanor with what many consider to be the persona non grata of society. Huggins displays an indomitableness of spirit, a strength of character, and a sense of compassion that comes only when one has known great pain.

Through his formal training in yoga and meditation, Huggins finds a new freedom that not only will sustain him but will also cause a ripple effect. It is one that will be felt years after he is released, and consequently will touch and renew thousands of lives.

I met Huggins in 2016 when he walked into our prison, one of the oldest maximum- security prisons in Pennsylvania, as part of a two hundred-hour yoga instructor training course he was leading. He told me that real freedom was a choice and that it entailed more than just not being in prison.

During my training, I experienced a peace and freedom that went far beyond anything I had ever experienced. Huggins became my teacher, guide, and mentor, reminding me that my life was not to be defined by external forces. I am grateful and forever indebted to Huggins and his team for giving me the tools to cut off the shackles, hold my head up high, and breathe freely and with a purpose.

Peace, joy, surrender, true self.

– Gabriel

Preface

They came into my cell and woke me at about 3 a.m. I knew it was coming. They'd made me pack my things a day and a half earlier. For a day I'd been without anything—not a toothbrush, book, or change of underwear. Just the green jumpsuit I was sleeping in.

I had been bracing myself for this, wondering if I could find the inner strength to survive Diesel Therapy. I knew this trip would mean an end of my five weeks in the hell that was the Federal Detention Center in Philadelphia, and from what I'd heard from the other inmates and even the prison counselor, pretty much wherever I might be going had to be better than the Philly FDC.

I was taken to a holding area where we were stripped out of our uniforms, searched, processed, and made to put on a blue paper jumpsuit. We were shackled, wrists to waist and ankles together so only baby steps were possible. Any tighter and the cold, hard metal would have ripped my skin or cut off circulation.

After waiting in a cold, underground bus depot, we were herded onto a bus. For some reason I thought it might be safer in the front, near the guard. Although he had a gun—several guns—I felt he was less of a threat than the angry men who were my fellow passengers. One prisoner was already going crazy, yelling and kicking.

When I had last spoken to my brother Larry, he said our brother Bob probably had only days left to live. Now while I was in transit, I would be out of touch with my family and no one would know where I was to let me know when he died. Would I be allowed a furlough to go to the funeral? I had little reason to hope the prison authorities might show me that small mercy. After all, I had been shackled and taken away right after my sentencing.

And all for a misdemeanor.

"St. Michael," they had called me as a kid. If my high school yearbook had an award for *Least Likely to go to Prison*, I'd have won it.

Now I was on a prison bus headed to whatever facility that powers far away had deemed would be my home for the next eight months.

The prestige I once had because of my Wharton MBA and as a company's CEO meant nothing here. To the men with the guns, I was no different from the drug dealers, gang members, and murderers with whom I shared this ride, some of whom were heading for long stretches in maximum-security federal penitentiaries. I could only hope my atypical white-collar crime would let me do my time in a prison camp—the days of the famous Club Feds were long gone—but at least I might not spend the better part of the next year in a place as bad as the FDC I'd just left. The shock of receiving a prison term at all for a misdemeanor, then being immediately taken directly from the courtroom to prison was surreal enough, so I was not about to make any predictions about the prison conditions.

In the predawn darkness, the bus pulled out on a journey, the final stop and timetable of which were a mystery to me. There was no point in asking anyone; even if they knew, they weren't going to tell me.

One thing was certain: it was going to be a long day, the first of many to follow. I could only hope my yoga training would give me the strength to survive this journey and whatever challenges lay beyond it. I knew about yoga "off the mat." Yoga in shackles, on a cold bus to an unknown destination, would put all of my lessons to a major test.

After layovers lasting from hours to days in Fort Dix, Manhattan, and Brooklyn, the gates of Lewisburg Federal Penitentiary swung open and the bus drove through. This was the ancient fortress that had housed Al Capone, John Gotti, Jimmy Hoffa, the World Trade Center bombers, and some of the gangsters depicted in the movie *Goodfellas*. Was this to be my home? I could only hope that number 60419066 wouldn't be called—begging me by name to disembark.

Chapter One
St. Michael

A pleaser pleases everyone but themselves.

My middle-class, Irish-Catholic upbringing couldn't have foretold the course my life would chart, in either its highs or lows. Not my rise to CEO or my fall to inmate, or leaving the corporate world to bring yoga to people in crisis.

I was born in 1957 in the Philadelphia suburb of Drexel Hill. Already on the scene were my brothers Bob and Larry; after me came Brendan and Mary. Five children seems like a huge family now, but for a Catholic family of the era, ours was not atypical, and many families who went to our church had many more kids than that.

Ours was the typical television family of the 1950s and '60s. Dad was a World War II vet who now lived the American dream, going from a poor upbringing to use the G.I. Bill to go to college. My mom kept house while he worked a white-collar job. Mom eventually went to work years later, after her children were at least in their teens.

Dad worked long hours for General Electric, and if he wasn't home by seven, we'd have dinner without him. He regretted all of the missed baseball games and concerts and family time that working cost him. He wasn't around that much, and if we got in trouble, Mom still gave us the cliché threat of that era: "Wait until your father gets home!"

About age seven, I started piano lessons and loved playing music, but the nun who taught the lessons at school was brutal, smacking my hands with a ruler when I made a mistake, so my parents took me out of her lessons. I took private lessons for a while with an elderly neighbor who taught only a few chords and gave me little incentive to practice, so I quit. I wish I had stuck with it; maybe there wouldn't have been as long a gap in my music education.

I began school at the Catholic elementary school, just one block down the street. As an altar boy, I liked to be asked to serve at funerals, which would get me out of school for hours. We went to church as a family every Sunday, and I was very proud when I made my First Communion and Confirmation.

My parents called me "St. Michael" without a hint of sarcasm. They rarely said it around me, but my siblings would overhear them describing me that way to others, and my brothers and sister didn't resent it because it seemed true to them, too. There is a stereotype that the middle child is a "pleaser," wanting everyone to like him. I was the third of five children, and played that pleaser role perfectly. Ironically, my willingness to please and reluctance to rock the boat would later prove to be one of my greatest failings.

My brother Larry was the rebellious one. He once said, "Show me a rule, I'll break it. Show Mike a rule, he'll follow it." That made my legal problems even less likely and much more confusing to everyone.

Larry could charm people with his semi-bad boy demeanor. I could charm them with my pleasing personality, without crossing the line into being a cloying goody-two-shoes—as we used to call the brownnosers who worked a little too hard to curry favor with the nuns. Bob, the quiet one, was so much older than me that we never really hung out that much while growing up.

— — —

When I was in the seventh grade, my dad was transferred to a position in New York City, so we moved to Middletown, New Jersey. Dad mounted a basketball hoop on the telephone pole outside our house, and we used the street as our court, pausing the shirts-vs-skins games when a car needed to drive through. In my memory, it seemed those games went on all day and into the evening, only ending when darkness shut them down. We rotated players in and out, sometimes going in for dinner and coming out to rejoin the game later.

It was during those street basketball games that I really started on my spiritual path. Ed, my new best friend in Middletown, and I would have some pretty deep philosophical and religious discussions—especially for thirteen-year-olds. One day as we waited to join the next game, he asked me if I thought that he and his sister and his parents were going to hell. He and his family were Jewish.

I had a hard time grasping what was so horrible about Ed and his family that they should all suffer that fate, in spite of what the nuns at my school had taught me. His parents were nice people who were good friends of my parents. I couldn't tell him that I believed that. I still was St. Michael, attending mass, and going to confession, but I was already questioning my belief in a religion that was so rigid and excluded too many good people. We didn't use the term "spirituality" then, but it was certainly what I was thinking: that it's possible to be a good person without being a Catholic.

Life was pretty simple but ideal. Although not a superstar, the skills I honed in Little League earned me a spot on the high school baseball team. I was left-handed, a big advantage for a baseball player, and I was glad the nuns' attempt to convert me to being completely right-handed hadn't worked. I still write right-handed but play sports with my left. Mostly I played first base, a good spot for a sure-handed leftie, with an occasional stint in the outfield, and did well at the plate. I was good enough that I was always pushed ahead to the next league up, and in high school I made "All-County."

If my teacher in second grade had asked what I wanted to be when I grew up, I'm sure I'd have answered musician or baseball player and would never have said I wanted to be a CEO or president of a company. Certainly I would not have said "yogi." The only yogis I knew were Berra and Bear. If I had it all to do over again, I'd have had more faith in my dreams; I might have failed, but I'd have had more fun.

I wasn't the most popular kid in the high school, nor was I an outcast, so I was elected to student council. In addition to those duties and baseball, I periodically played piano in a band. We played a couple of high school dances, mainly doing Crosby, Stills, and Nash-style three- or four-part harmonies. Unfortunately, I can't sing at all. They gave me a microphone, but never turned it on, and for some songs I'd silently lip-synch what the other guys were singing. One crazy gimmick we had was that on a few songs, the bass player and I left our instruments and held our guitar player up by his feet while he played guitar upside down. It was a popular part of the act.

I never gave any serious thought to music as a career. For one thing, I wasn't that good—although I think with better teachers and more practice, I could have been. And although my parents never explicitly said it, there was an expectation that my siblings and I would all pursue more traditional and secure careers. Having been raised during the Depression, our parents were conscious of their kids having a safe financial path.

I was part of the concert committee in high school that picked Bruce Springsteen to perform for a class event. I can say that I hired "The Boss" when he was a local musician and still small-time enough to play a high school.

— — —

I got a summer job in the nearby town of Red Bank, which led to some of the most interesting moments of my life up to that point. I started as a busboy and rose to the job of waiter at the Molly Pitcher Inn, where I met not only some of the biggest name celebrities of the day, but also a coworker who eventually became my wife. I kept the job throughout my summers in college; it paid well and was interesting, in that most of the stars who performed at the nearby Garden State Art Center stayed or at least ate at the Molly Pitcher.

For a week, I was the personal waiter to George Burns and his entourage of eight or so people. One night during dinner I was giving Mr. Burns and his group some space while they ate. I had walked over to the large picture windows and was gazing down at the beautiful view of the Navesink River below. I heard his very distinctive voice next to me. "What are you looking at? Oh!" He noticed that also below me was the hotel's swimming pool, and lounging beside it were two very attractive young women in bikinis. He was probably in his '80s, but he smiled at me and asked, "What do you want to bet that I could get those young ladies to come up to my room?" Before I could even reply, he was gone, out the door and headed down the path to the pool, toying with his ever-present but rarely lit cigar as he went.

I watched as he talked with the women. A few minutes later, he was coming back up the path, a bathing beauty on each arm. He looked up at the window, smiled and waved at me.

The next day when I saw him, I said, "That was really good."

"Nothing happened. I'm too old for that sort of nonsense. I just get girls for my piano player. He gives me money, I give him girls," he said, with the trademark twinkle in his voice. He was as warm and charming a man as he seemed on TV.

Henny Youngman was also just what I expected, throwing out one-liners nonstop.

Me: "How would you like your steak?"

Youngman: "On a plate."

I could almost hear the rim shot after everything he said. His wife kept telling him to stop clowning. You'd think after however many years they'd been together that she'd have been used to his act, but I still found it amusing.

One summer, a new hire, Jenny, was assigned to my team. It was apparent that, in spite of what she had claimed on her application, she really didn't have much experience waiting tables. I kind of liked her from the start, so I covered for her and trained her as she learned on the job.

My first official date with Jenny was to see Springsteen play at the Stone Pony in Asbury Park. The Stone Pony is another great music venue that helped launch the career of Springsteen and several other local talents.

That fall, I returned to college at Villanova; ironically it was at a Catholic university, where I took another step away from being Catholic. In a comparative religions class, I saw the distinction between religion and spirituality; I had an awakening about nondualism, though I didn't know it was called that then. The idea that we could not separate ourselves from others, that we were not distinct from what was around us, was a notion that stuck with me.

After college, I landed a job at one of the giant accounting firms, Arthur Andersen. I passed the CPA exam and could have settled into life there, but was still grasping for something more—although I could not have begun to express what that might be. I just felt there should be more to life than this.

— — —

I had continued to date Jenny, and while I was at Andersen, we became engaged. But if I wanted to make partner, I would have to pay my dues in terms of long hours and a lot of travel, and she wasn't sure she wanted to be married to someone who was married to his job. I was also partying too much with my training team and she saw that as another concern, so after a few months, she broke off the engagement.

Losing Jenny woke me up to the life I had chosen. Did I really want to spend at least ten years keeping up this kind of pace before I'd make partner? In thinking about the path I was on, I realized something: I didn't want to be an accountant. Deciding to return to school and get a Master of Business Administration, I was accepted into the prestigious Wharton School of Business at the University of Pennsylvania.

It was great, since I would still be close to family, but I had seriously under-budgeted for living expenses, and with my younger siblings still in college, didn't feel right asking my parents for help.

The cheapest place I could find to live that first year of grad school was in a sober living house for men. Little did I know that this experience of sharing too small a space with too many men of questionable hygiene habits, some of whom had problems with drugs and other issues, would be schooling of a different sort. Some of the skills I learned there for tolerating others and living without many of the basic comforts of the modern world would come back to me when I was in prison years later.

Everyone in the house shared one bathroom down the hall. Not a good situation with the cleanest of guys, and certainly not fun with these housemates. We had no kitchen privileges, so I had a college dorm-sized refrigerator and a hot plate, and had to shop and cook accordingly. I learned to do a lot with a little, another talent that would serve me well in the federal pen.

My car had been run into by someone without insurance, and I didn't have enough coverage to be able to have it repaired, so I was also without a car. That meant long, and sometimes very cold, bicycle rides from the campus through a crime-ridden part of town. When it was really cold, I'd splurge and spend the money on a SEPTA ticket, but bikes technically weren't allowed on the trains, so I had to try to smuggle it on. It was far from the Ivy-League life of many of my fellow students, who were driving their imported sports cars to class.

The major aspiration of many of my classmates seemed to become multimillionaires. They didn't seem to particularly care how. But this was the heyday of Drexel Burnham and their ilk and most of my classmates had Wall Street dreams and dollar signs in their eyes. I wanted to make something in addition to money and had a vague idea of how to do that, perhaps in manufacturing.

In 1984, I got my MBA. As I saw my life on a better path, or at least a more secure one, Jenny reentered my life. We had loosely stayed in touch during the breakup, and one evening she called me, distraught about the horrible day she'd had and just needing a friendly shoulder on which to cry. After she calmed down, we ended up on the phone for hours talking about everything under the sun, including what had gone wrong between us.

I had just started dating someone else, but the long heart-to-heart with Jenny rekindled my feelings for her and we decided to give each other another try.

Decades later, when our marriage ended, I read that a broken engagement should be taken as a huge red flag, and those marriages that occur after a breakup rarely last. But at the time, things seemed off to a good start. I got a job with General Mills near Minneapolis and my bride and I set off to our happy new lives together.

8

Chapter Two
The Huggins Principle

The Huggins Principle: the inverse relationship between my income and "status" to my state of happiness.

After a few job-related relocations, Jenny and I settled into life in the Boston suburbs, where we ended up staying for twelve years. I started as a financial analyst for a jewelry manufacturing company. I was supposed to keep the numbers straight, but I quickly got more responsibility and moved into larger positions until I became vice president of manufacturing, reporting directly to the CEO. I found I liked seeing things get made more than I just liked crunching numbers. The one thing I didn't like was the travel; the company did much of its business overseas, and I fell into a pattern that would go on the rest of my corporate career—being away from home too much of the time.

When I traveled to the Far East, my boss had wanted me to go with him to shady massage parlors and other places I didn't want to go. At another company where I worked, we fired an employee for sending pornographic emails. I wouldn't tolerate that sort of thing. My straight-laced approach to things may have marked me as a prude and a stickler for the rules, but it also made my eventual downfall even more ironic.

Jenny and I had one daughter and adopted another. Erin and Maria were wonderful additions to our lives, but with the arrival of the kids, Jenny and I also very slowly started going in different directions. Jenny put all her attention into being a mother, while I put energy into my career, and I began to realize that we really didn't have a lot in common any longer. Or maybe we never did.

With the girls, of course we partook in the usual traditions with Santa and the Easter Bunny, but as Irish as our family was, I invented a mischief leprechaun who would sneak into the girls' room the night before St. Patrick's Day, make a mess, and play pranks. He also left candy and money. Once Maria was old enough to realize her parents were really the leprechaun, she took over playing pranks and eventually shifted it to April Fool's Day, although between March 17 and April, any sort of practical joke was possible. One day I went outside to get in my car to go to work and found it completely encased in plastic wrap.

I did a lot of the cooking and wanted to make it fun. One year for Thanksgiving, I dressed the large turkey in an aluminum foil bikini, so when it was done cooking, it had tan lines as though it had just come from the beach. When we lived in Massachusetts and lobster was readily available, I'd often let the crustaceans loose to run around the floor, to the delight and fright of the girls—like the scene in the Woody Allen movie *Annie Hall*.

We had a pretty good life, and I wanted a career path that would ensure it would continue.

In 1994, the man who had preceded me in my position at the jewelry company offered me a position as assistant to the Chief Operating Officer of a medical device company in Paoli, Pennsylvania. In addition to its being a good opportunity to continue to climb the corporate ladder, it had the added advantage of being close to Philadelphia and to my parents and some of my siblings, and we'd also be closer to Jenny's family in New Jersey.

One day in Massachusetts, some neighborhood kids set up a ramp in the street and were using it as a jump for their bikes. I was rollerblading, and for some reason thought it would be a good idea to take the jump on my skates. I landed hard on my butt. After everyone, myself and daughters included, had a good laugh, I realized I was more hurt than I first thought. The injury meant that I couldn't do much of my regular routine at the gym, and I wasn't happy.

A friend recommended that I try yoga as a gentle way of rehabilitating my back. The instructor for my first class, Colleen DeVirgiliis, was new to teaching, but she made it very welcoming and appealing. We bonded immediately. She was to become an important part of my journey into yoga and into myself.

— — —

When I started, I treated yoga more like a sport. Like many people who start doing yoga, I was more interested in learning the poses to get the physical benefits and didn't care to know much about the spiritual or emotional benefits. It was great for my back, and at some point I just started feeling better physically and mentally.

For those unfamiliar with the practice, there are over one thousand yoga poses, developed over five thousand years. Most practices utilize a few dozen of the most popular—pigeon, crow, tree, happy baby, downward dog—some of which are much more difficult than others. Some practice yoga for years without ever mastering many of the more challenging poses. An instructor guides the students through the poses, prompting them to shift from one into the next.

Yoga soon became my chosen form of exercise, and several mornings a week I'd stop by the gym on my way to work. On business trips, I'd often seek out a yoga studio near my hotel or just do my own routine in my room.

— — —

The company that had lured me back to Eastern Pennsylvania was Synthes. It was a large company with thousands of employees around the world, manufacturing and selling a variety of products that were classified by the Food and Drug Administration (FDA) as "medical devices." These included implants and screws, plates, rods, and cements that repaired bones—products that allowed doctors to save limbs after accidents.

A book could be written just about the odd corporate culture at Synthes, primarily created and embodied by the owner and CEO. And several more books could be written about the legal issues that were to become my undoing. There is no sound bite or elevator version of the story that could begin to do justice to the complexities of what really happened. This would later present a problem in the press, in court, in prison, and beyond. It took more than a few minutes to explain the mess and a few minutes into any summation, I'd watch people's brows furrow and their eyes glaze over: they weren't getting the nuances, nor did most people particularly want to. Even those who did want to understand had a hard time doing so. In prison, it was spread around that I was in for some sort of medical fraud. That was not what I did, but sometimes I didn't have the time or energy to set people straight.

There were parts of the job that I found exciting: here I was, a kid from relatively humble beginnings, traveling the world on a corporate jet, wining and dining CEOs.

In addition to the perks of the jet and a nice salary, I was drawn to Synthes due to my love of manufacturing. At times, I'd spend extended periods at our large manufacturing facility in Colorado, where I got to know and love the people and the products. Working the warehouse with enthusiasm, I assembled and checked orders, jumping in and filling gaps wherever they were in the process—and subsequently earning the respect of everyone there. There was no job that I felt was beneath me. It also helped me to learn the entire manufacturing process and fully understand what the company did. But the novelty and the perks wear off quickly, and it can be draining to always be on the go—especially when there was no end in sight for sudden, open-ended trips. It's tough to be a good parent or husband from 1,700 miles away.

I was on a very fast track at Synthes and maybe I was getting too swept up in the high life, but more gaps in my relationship with Jenny were starting to appear. Several top execs got invited to fly to Switzerland for a big meeting, and I was able to bring my Jenny. It was her first time flying business class, but instead of reveling in the comfort the way I did, it seemed to make her uncomfortable. The trip, a work retreat in the mountains, involved a good deal of business, but there were also many dinners, parties, and social activities. I loved it. She hated it. She didn't like to blend business and social lives. Rather than succumbing to the pressure to make small talk with people she didn't know, Jenny would often retreat to our room and leave me to go to the cocktail hours alone. I realized we had different likes and expectations for my career and for our shared future.

But with each higher position at the company, the stresses grew correspondingly greater, and I was traveling more than ever. After just using yoga as exercise, I found myself opening up to the deeper aspects of yoga—wanting to concentrate on relaxing my body and focus on breathing as a way to escape from the increasing strain I was feeling at work. What I started as a low-impact workout was becoming a refuge of mental quiet time in the whirlwind of my life.

As at other companies, on business trips it was pretty typical for the guys to hang out in the hotel bar or some nearby watering hole in the evenings. That hadn't been my scene in a long time. Instead, I'd seek out a local yoga studio or do my own meditations and routines in my hotel room.

Even before I got into yoga—a practice that changed my mind-set about a lot of things—I managed people differently than many corporate executives. I was much less autocratic and I respected everyone. I treated the custodians and the workers on the factory floor the same way I treated the president of a division. I tried to find the right people for key positions and trusted them to do their jobs properly—this should be axiomatic in business, but Synthes's owner could come on strong at times, often testing people and pushing their buttons. I earned the loyalty and respect of pretty much everyone in the company, many of whom rallied to my defense when things went bad. At times after the legal problems began, I wondered if I had taken a more hands-on or micromanaging approach, maybe some of the problems could have been avoided. I had middle-of-the-night doubts, but I also tried not to dwell on something that I couldn't travel back in time and change.

— — —

Because the products and techniques to use these devices were so technical, the company (along with all of our competitors) hired reps to instruct the surgical teams in the use of the products. Being the expert on the products meant our reps were on call, as a surgeon would be. They'd get 2 a.m. phone calls to rush to the hospital—someone had been injured in an accident, and to save that victim's leg one of our implants was necessary. The rep would be in the O.R., to make sure the product was available and that the surgeon had the necessary instruments to perform the surgery. It felt good to be part of something that helped people, and in some cases, saved lives.

Initially, I had nothing to do with the sales side. My job was in manufacturing and operations, but after I was promoted to VP of Operations, I had more people answering to me. I was enjoying the job and seeing the valuable work we were doing—jewelry never saved lives.

As I grew into higher positions, I had the power and confidence to let my methods influence the way things went on a larger scale at work. It was a good feeling to know that I was helping make the corporate culture more accepting, and I think we were able to keep some good people because of that.

I also tried to have fun at work. We formed a band at Synthes called the Spinal Chords. I played the keyboards, and we did covers of rock standards, including "Proud Mary" and "American Pie," but we changed the lyrics so they were about bone surgery. To the tune of Marvin Gaye's "I Heard It Through the Grapevine," we sang about some of our new products:

Ooh, I bet you're wondering how I know
about your plans to help me grow.
With some systems I've never seen before.
You will sure help me sell much more.
It took me by surprise I must say, when I found out yesterday
Don't you know that...

We got products through the pipeline.
Pangea and ProDisc, you are now mine.
So many products through the pipeline.
Oh, and I'm just about to lose my mind.

Maybe only people in the business really appreciated the jokes, but our target audience sure did. One year, we gave a CD of our music to surgeons we sold to, and were surprised and pleased when we found that it became popular to play in the operating room. Many of the types of procedures in which our products were used required hours of tedious surgery, and most surgeons played music in the operating room.

On business trips, instead of golfing or participating in other corporate type events, I would hike with small groups of employees—or at my own expense, take them sailing on the Chesapeake and get to know them on a deeper level. Most people saw me as serious around the office, and I think they were surprised at how their boss could completely cut loose and get into music or sailing.

At one point, I saw enough promise in the growing company that when there was an opening in another department and my brother Larry was looking to change jobs, I recommended that he apply. It wasn't awkward for either of us and didn't violate company policy because it was in a different area, and he didn't report to me either directly or indirectly. The FDA investigation came to his section, and therefore his attention, before it came to mine. In the medical device industry, everyone gets used to having the FDA look over their shoulders, so he didn't think it was too worrisome at the time.

I was promoted to Chief Operating Officer of the U.S. division and eventually became the global president of the spine business. At this point, I felt I could make significant changes in the way people managed and treated each other. I had read *The Four Agreements*, a small and rather simple book written, appropriately enough, by a Mexican surgeon, Dr. Don Miguel Ruiz. The book had nothing to do with surgery or medicine. It was based on ancient Toltec teachings and was really quite simple: 1) Be impeccable with your word; 2) Don't take anything personally*; 3) Don't make assumptions; 4) Always do your best.

* The second one was hard to keep in mind as the storm got closer and closer to engulfing me.

I handed out copies of the book to the senior team I was now managing, and we spent several hours talking about *The Four Agreements* and how this would change the way we dealt with each other, our customers, and everyone in our lives. Of course the book expanded on all of these, but I kept the Four Agreements on a small card that I kept among my business cards, as a reminder.

Our Senior VP of Sales was successful by following his gut intuition, yet I wanted and needed systems and numbers. To reconcile the two styles, I brought in a psychologist, who did profiles of each of our top people and how we could work together better. We gave everyone a Myers-Briggs test, and through our different styles found ways to communicate better. I hoped this would set the tone for the business and flow down to everyone in the division. Although these sorts of things were becoming common at many companies, they weren't yet standard at Synthes. Much of what I did (and what people said made me effective in my job) was to provide a calming counterbalance to the big boss's sometimes irrational moments.

Still, in many ways I marched to the beat of a different drummer. At one sales meeting, there was a golf outing planned. I had played golf but never really enjoyed it, so I decided to offer a yoga class as an alternative. I thought I might get half a dozen people to skip the golf course in favor of downward dog, but to my amazement, about forty of the 350 people who were at the event signed up for the yoga class. I was to find that there were a lot of closet yoga fans in the corporate world. People would say, "I hit the gym before work," or, "I'm going to the gym at lunchtime," but thought there was something too new-agey about admitting it was yoga they were doing at the gym.

— — —

Despite the excitement, perks, and stroking of the ego that came with the job, I started to tire from the grind of constant travel, meetings, and pressure to deliver results. The highs seemed to come less frequently, and the lows were coming faster and lasting longer. Perhaps the accumulation of almost thirty years of working in high-pressure positions was taking a toll on me. Or perhaps my yoga practice was allowing me to see and feel things from a different perspective.

By 2007, I was burned out and getting signs that things weren't right in my life. My best friend passed away; I had worked with him at Synthes, and we often socialized outside of work. His loss and a few other things seemed to pile up, and I wasn't feeling comfortable in my own skin any longer. My marriage, my job, everything seemed to not fit as well as it once did. I was getting more seriously into yoga and meditation, and both my body and my mind were telling me it was time for a change. I decided to leave Synthes.

Although it factored very little in my decision to leave, in retrospect, many people suspected that I could see the storm clouds coming from the government's investigation of Synthes. The truth is, though I knew about the investigation, I was not yet a target of the probe and thought the issue would be handled with no major fallout. I couldn't have been more wrong.

The government was looking into allegations that some doctors were using one of our products off-label, and that some of our sales reps and sales manager may have been aware of this use and not acting appropriately to curtail it. Pharmaceutical companies are often the targets of similar investigations and pay a fine, pledge to fix the problem, and that is the end of it. Even if this investigation went anywhere, I never thought it would reach up to me. Doctors are allowed to prescribe or use what they like for whatever purpose, but companies that make those drugs or devices are not allowed to even imply that the product is good for any purpose other than those for which it was specifically approved by the FDA.

When I left Synthes, I did some consulting while I explored going back to school to get my PhD in business. I liked the idea of going into teaching, as my father had done later in his career—a move that made him happier and more fulfilled than the corporate world ever did.

But the path back into academia was looking too long and twisted. As much as I wanted out of the corporate world, a whisper in my other ear was saying that I was supposed to keep climbing the ladder. When I was offered the position as chief executive officer of another medical company, I took it. There was an expectation that if a promotion and a bigger title came your way, you were supposed to take them.

The first voice was telling me it was a mistake to keep returning to the C-suite (CEO, CFO, COO) when it had begun to feel more and more like the wrong place to be. Instead of the Peter Principle—rather than hitting my level of incompetence—I had risen to my level of unhappiness. I was the embodiment of what I came to call the Huggins Principle, something I had seen time and time again among family and friends and coworkers: Many people found it much harder to go back down the ladder to a more comfortable rung than to keep climbing to more precarious and worrisome heights. I had seen many talented engineers, salespeople, and accountants rise to a management position where they were miserable and much less effective in their new positions than in their old ones.

The frying pan wasn't even warm at Synthes when I jumped and found myself in a hot fire. Rather than listening to my gut and following my heart, I had joined another medical device company. My ego overwhelmed my intuition. Almost immediately, I started having disagreements with the board on a variety of topics. From the day I started, something told me I'd made a great mistake. The company was based in Paris but had a small distribution operation in Florida, so I was traveling more than ever—about 90 percent of the time. I disliked the way the company had been run prior to my arrival, the additional time away from my family, and the feeling that I was in the wrong place at the wrong time. The only thing keeping me happy and sane was my yoga.

Meanwhile, the FDA's investigation of Synthes now had grown to involve the Department of Justice. In April 2009, I received a grand jury subpoena and became aware that there was the very real possibility that criminal charges could be brought against Synthes and some individuals who worked there—including me.

I didn't want to bring any harm to my current employer, and so I arranged with its senior management a plan to announce my resignation.

— — —

While I was becoming embroiled in the criminal investigation, my oldest brother, Bob, fell sick. It was a shock—Bob had always been in such great shape. He ran 10Ks and marathons on a regular basis for years. Then he shattered his ankle in an accident—he ran in all weather and got caught miles from home during an ice storm. He slipped on the ice and went down in a ditch, destroying his ankle. He had major reconstructive surgery—using Synthes parts, ironically, although this was a few years before I would go to work for the company.

Bob tried everything to attempt to rehabilitate the leg but nothing worked; he would never run again. He tried to stay attached to the sport by starting a company that produced races, but he found it hard to be around the sport he loved and not be able to run. He came down hard from a lifetime of runner's highs.

He used to come over to our house and watch *The X-Files* every Sunday evening. We'd make an event of it—make popcorn and set up the chairs theater-style so everyone had a good view of the TV. Bob would often bring *X-Files* action figures or toys and remind us that "the truth was out there." Erin and Maria would laugh as he pointed out some of the cheesier special effects or plotlines. He also got us to watch *Mystery Science Theater 3000*, and he would join with Crow and Tom Servo in mocking the bad movies, much to the delight of my daughters. His logical, scientific mind pointed out inconsistencies in the plots of both *X-Files* and *MST 3000*, which we all—including Bob—found hilarious considering the absurd premises of the shows.

All through their childhoods, he was great with my daughters. He'd take them shopping, and he loved Black Friday sales. But after his running days were over, it took some of the spark out of his life. It was hard to watch him sink into depression.

One day Bob collapsed, resulting in a hospital stay. After a second collapse, he began a slow, downhill slide from a host of physical ailments, which kept piling one on top of another. He eventually had to have his foot amputated.

My brother Larry and I lived closest to Bob, so it was clear that the two of us would have to start checking up on our oldest brother. Since I wasn't working and had more time for this, Bob became primarily my responsibility. We moved him in with us and my family tried to nurse him back to health, but at some point it became apparent to all of us that he didn't want to get better—a fact that was incredibly hard on everyone.

On the legal front, after much soul searching, in July of 2009, I signed an agreement pleading guilty that I was a "responsible corporate officer" for misconduct that existed at lower levels of the company. Three other executives at Synthes made the same deal with the government.

The misdemeanor exists because the medical device industry, like the pharmaceutical industry, is highly regulated by the FDA, and the Supreme Court of the United States has held that high-level officers of companies regulated by the FDA can be held responsible for "public welfare" offenses, even if they did not: intend to do anything wrong, or knowingly do anything wrong, or directly participate in the misconduct.

I was surprised to learn that such officers can be charged and not just fined, but actually jailed if something goes wrong on their watch. The justification for the law is that those corporate officers should have known and done something to stop it. I had three divisions, plus manufacturing and administration reporting to me, with seven direct reports and over 1,500 employees.

There were a host of potentially worse charges and, given the way the case against us was inflated, taking the plea agreement seemed the best option for all of us.

I, along with the other three executives charged, had to agree to the deal, or we would all stand trial together. As part of the plea deal, we knew we could each face jail—at least theoretically. I was prepared for the worst, but the notion that someone would go to prison for a misdemeanor that did not even require proof of knowledge or intent was hardly commonplace. The lawyers for one of the other defendants made a big point of arguing in the sentencing documents they filed that there was no prior instance of someone going to federal prison for the misdemeanor offense to which we pleaded guilty. As it turned out, the judge did not take kindly to that argument. We could be the example to other execs.

The plea was entered and now I had to await sentencing. I settled into what was to be the most agonizing period of my life to date: purgatory.

Chapter Three
Purgatory

*The certainty of uncertainty removes the safety net
to provide the freedom to face our fears.*

Purgatory, as described in Catholic catechism, refers to the period after someone dies while they await judgment and possibly entry into heaven. It is also known as "limbo," which is exactly the state my life had become as I awaited judgment. While this unknown outcome hung over me, there wasn't much I could do. The legal wrangling was taking up much of my time, and I was devoting a good deal of time to looking after Bob, with help from Larry and his wife, Sharon.

Months of this waiting dragged into years. Everything seemed in an excruciating downward spiral: Bob had his good periods, but was clearly on a decline; the outcome of the legal problems didn't look good; and my marriage was also deteriorating.

For a long time I thought the distance I felt from Jenny was due to traveling so much and working so hard. Now that those distractions were no longer present, what was my excuse?

Had I changed that much? Maybe I hadn't really changed at all. Maybe I was just finally accepting who I was always meant to be. I had pretended to be the person Jenny wanted to marry, the person I was expected to be for her and everyone else in my life, but not the person I wanted to be. It would be wrong to say I was never happy as an adult—I was. I had moments of great joy with Jenny, my daughters, the rest of my family, and friends. I had career highs and other accomplishments that made me very proud. But something was missing. I wanted something more. I had also done so much to please other people, but I wanted to do more to feel like I was really making a difference—and really pleasing myself for perhaps the first time in my life.

I had watched friends' marriages fall apart, and they usually had a major cause—someone had been unfaithful, one of the partners had an out-of-control spending or drinking problem, or there was some other clear-cut reason for their separation. In the case of Jenny and me, it was nothing in particular. A lot of little things, but nothing big that I could articulate. In a way, this made our struggles more difficult because I could hardly explain things to myself, let alone to others.

Starting to think seriously about divorcing or at least separating from Jenny, I went to talk things out with Larry. I always marveled at how happy he and Sharon seemed to be together. In that heart-to-heart with him, he told me, "I'm as in love with her today as the day I married her." I almost wanted him to say that no one could expect to be all that happy in a marriage after several decades and that I should just deal with it. Instead, he told me that he and Sharon still were very, very happy. They still did everything as a team. Larry said, "There is, or should be, more to a relationship than just putting up with the other person."

However, I didn't have a lot of time to think clearly about Jenny, as Bob and the legal woes both worsened.

— — —

My fellow defendants and I knew we shouldn't talk to journalists or issue any kind of statements, and in the meantime we were getting ripped apart in both the Philadelphia press and, to some degree, the national media. Before I was in this situation, whenever I read a news story with that damning line, "And John Smith declined to comment…" I wondered what the guy was hiding. We were already the bad guys in this story, and anything we said was likely to get twisted. Every time a story about our case ran, there were numerous factual errors, but trying to straighten it out would have taken more newspaper column inches than any publication was likely to grant us. Our guilty pleas only made it easier for us to be convicted in the court of public opinion: after all, we had said we were guilty of *something*. But we were not guilty of the host of accusations we were charged with by the media.

The prosecutors made it sound as though we held secret meetings during which we had plotted to risk human lives for corporate profit. Nothing even remotely like that ever occurred. It never once crossed my mind to try to cover up or lie my way out of this situation, but it was clear that the judge thought otherwise. Allegedly, the company acted out of greed, but Synthes never profited or even attempted to profit from what was done.

— — —

During this time, I continued practicing yoga and trying to do some introspection, which I had seemingly been running from most of my life. While I had been so busy, it was easy for me to run from the things that had bothered me for so long. Now I had time and no place to run.

I started reading more spiritual books and seeing things differently. There are a lot of Buddhist principles embedded in yoga, and although I was not becoming a Buddhist, examining things from a very different perspective made me decide that I could not remain an active Catholic. Bob was still very Catholic, and we discussed the similarities and differences between the religion in which we had been raised and Buddhism. I told him that I preferred the Buddhist view because it never got caught up in the political hierarchy of a "church," which seemed to get in the way of its message of love and compassion. The concepts of love and honesty were instilled in me, if not always practiced by the church itself.

No one in my family had ever been divorced, and if things didn't work out with Jenny, I was sure my family would be very disappointed. My Irish-Catholic guilt had me feeling bad that I was hurting my parents. Strange how much the child in me wanted to please my mom and dad, even though I was an adult with grown children of my own.

I already felt horrible for my parents. They were about to lose two sons: Bob, permanently, and me, possibly temporarily, but in a way, my situation was harder to explain. I could barely explain it myself. Knowing how proud my parents were of me, I could only imagine the awkward moment that would come when one of their friends or further-flung relatives would ask, "What's Mike up to?" As much sadder as Bob's illness was, it was also much easier for them to tell their friends about.

One huge asset Bob and I had during our parallel, but very different journeys into darkness, was our family. There was never any doubt in my mind or in my siblings' that if I was in crisis or Bob was, the entire family would rally to the cause to be as supportive as they could in any way possible. There is grief in losing a child to a serious illness, but there is not shame. Although my parents were completely supportive and understanding of my circumstances, I know there had to be some awkwardness when they talked about me.

Never one to sit still, I I often became too involved in too many things even as a child, to the point that my parents would caution me to slow down. I was busy with Bob and answering legal questions, but I kept adding more activities to my plate, including teaching a graduate course at the local Penn State University branch campus.

— — —

As I dove deeper into yoga and had the time to do it, I decided to become a full-fledged yoga teacher, surprising some friends and many of the people I encountered in my training. Most of my fellow students were fresh out of college, and here I was at age fifty-two, embarking on a path that not many Wharton MBAs and former CEOs were pursuing. For someone who had always tried to fit and conform, it was liberating to buck the norm for a change.

Yoga teacher training gave me the internal strength to cope with the many other changes that were swirling around me. There are really two elements to yoga: the physical and the spiritual. At its most fulfilling, yoga should be a perfect blending of both, one element complimenting the other in yin and yang. While stretching into or holding an awkward pose, it often takes full concentration to avoid losing balance. Having to focus on the body makes it impossible to still be stuck on unproductive thoughts. Shutting off the brain to think only about the body is amazingly liberating.

Life is always about change, but I was getting yanked far out of my comfort zone, and I hoped to be able to control some of those changes instead of just being battered by the storm. As any sailor knows, it's useless to fight against the wind: you have to partner with the wind to get anywhere and not get ripped apart. The biggest upheavals were things over which I had no control. I couldn't change the wind; I could only adjust my sails and prepare to meet the storm.

— — —

There has always been that debate of what makes people who they are—nature or nurture? Bob and I were products of the same genes and same environment, and yet so completely different. I was outgoing and eager to try new things. He had always been shy. Without being antisocial, he also wasn't big into making friends or dating, and at some point he had decided he was too set in his ways to think anyone might want him. He was a bit of a hoarder and lived on his own terms. Because of the age gap and the lack of common interests, we had never spent a great deal of time together. Now, while spending time with my brother, I was learning a lot about life and how different people think.

Fate had almost forced Bob and me to spend time together. At first I set out to "fix" Bob; I kept trying to tell him what to do to get better. This led to many arguments and he started to resent my meddling. At some point, I decided to follow what yoga had been trying to teach me and what I had been resisting—to just let things be as they are: accept them.

If Bob had a stronger will to live he might have overcome those difficulties, but he didn't want to save himself or want anyone else to save him—as though I or anyone else could. It was a lesson that would be repeated so many times with men I'd meet in prison, though their struggles may have been completely different from Bob's. I had to remember that while I could offer my help, that help had to take the form of my guiding them on a path, not forcing them down a path, or carrying them down a path. Once I backed off with Bob, I found a friend. We were able to compare notes on our struggles and somehow find a way to laugh about them.

Meanwhile, things with Jenny were getting worse. She and I were at our vacation home in Wildwood, New Jersey, and one day we had a big argument. I knew if I didn't leave, I would say something I'd regret, so I got on my bicycle and rode for a while before finding a quiet spot near the water to practice yoga and meditate. I'd had small moments of enlightenment doing yoga, but for the first time—and at a moment when I very much needed it—I had my first major epiphany.

I had heard from a few fellow practitioners, and would hear it many times in future classes, that someone had a breakthrough of some sort while practicing yoga. Some people had told me that even in their very first session, they'd had a glimpse of the power of yoga. Other people went for years without ever achieving that moment of extreme clarity. It's hard to explain to someone who has never had one of those yoga highs. It could take the form of looking deep inside to see a part of themselves they had never seen before, or looking outward to gain an insight of the world they had never known existed. Some people compared this to certain drug experiences; never having done drugs, I couldn't be sure. The advantage of yoga was that it wasn't artificial chemicals producing this change of consciousness; it was the body and mind's own catalysts that produced the shift.

I needed to take more control of my life and needed to be alone to do that. I rode back to the house, nervous about what I had to do, but also completely at peace with my decision. I told Jenny I needed space and that we should separate, at least temporarily, while I sorted things out. I am still not sure couching it as "temporary" wasn't just to assuage her feelings or my guilt, but even as I was proposing it, I knew deep down that it was likely permanent; the insight I had just had seemed to make that clear. After twenty-eight years, I just couldn't pretend to be happy in my marriage any longer. With all of the other things facing me, I didn't have the energy for the pretense or the fight.

In some very odd way, my facing possible prison time and having my reputation torn apart in the press helped free me to make this decision. My integrity had always meant so much to me, and it was a bitter thing to see myself accused of horrible things in print that I wasn't even being accused of by the Department of Justice. It was time to let go of the ego that said that others' opinions of me were more important than being true to myself.

One of the strange juxtapositions of events was that I had so much extra time to volunteer, that the local chapter of the United Way gave me their service award. How was this the same horrible person who was being tried and convicted in the media?

I was letting go of some things, and starting to hold others tighter. I wanted to reassure my daughters that no matter what happened between their mother and me, I didn't want my relationship with the girls to change—except possibly to make it better and make up for the father-daughter time we had lost to years of work and travel. My older daughter, Erin, was living in Washington, DC, and when Jenny chose to remain at our place in New Jersey, it was now just Maria and me living at home. Maria and I decided to pursue our personal training certificates, so we got to spend a lot of time together commuting to the classes and studying together. It was another bonding experience—the memory of which would comfort me at lonely times in prison.

When a couple splits up, their friends tend to pick sides, so I lost some of my support group. Perhaps my fretting over my legal issues made me not very good company, but while some friends stayed close and even got closer, other friends distanced themselves, and I found myself getting fewer invitations to do things. I found myself drinking a lot. I wasn't going out to bars; I was just sitting home downing a few gin and tonics or rum and Diet Cokes each evening, while watching historical documentaries on TV. It was a strange contrast from dealing with stress in one of the healthiest ways possible—practicing yoga and going to yoga trainings by day—to handling it in one of the worst ways possible—with alcohol every evening. I never drove drunk. I just sat at home, got drunk alone, and went to bed.

— — —

An unwelcome hobby that consumed much of my time now was dealing with legal entanglements. It seemed like every day I had to address some aspect of the case as it took twists and turns, each one seeming to cause another issue.

I was now into my second year of waiting, and each time we seemed to be getting closer to a sentencing date, the possibility of time behind bars would rear its ugly head and I'd start to worry. Catholics may not have quite the inborn level of impending doom that many of my Jewish friends seemed to have, but we papists are a close second; maybe it has something to do with how we were taught that after all Christ had suffered for us, we should just offer up our own suffering to him. It was hard to shake the feeling that some dreadful fate was just over the horizon. Like a long hike or sailing trip, every time I thought my destination was in sight, I realized I had a long way to go. Never having been through anything like this, I didn't have a compass to help me navigate or a calendar by which to mark time, and I was left at times staring off at a frightening nothingness.

Maybe I was fixating too much on prisons, but it had me imagining what guys on death row must endure. I had never been to jail or even visited one before. I had not given much thought to prisons or prisoners. It's like so many things in life: if there is no direct impact on our own lives, how much attention do we pay to it? Everyone knows Alzheimer's disease exists, but does anyone try to learn about its progression or possible treatments until it strikes someone close?

What little thought I had ever given to prison could be pretty well summed up in the phrase, "if you do the crime, you gotta do the time." I imagined every possible scenario for what prison would be like— maybe it would be Club Fed, where I could play tennis and eat fresh kale from a salad bar. Maybe it would be the *Shawshank Redemption*, only worse. I knew the truth likely lay between my fears and hopes, but at times I could delude myself into one extreme or the other. It was hard not to dwell on the prospects. The only place I seemed free of the nagging worry was on the yoga mat. My little 18-by-60-inch piece of peace.

— — —

When I was COO or CEO, my ego liked being in charge. When I first got into yoga, I had that same ego investment. I was more into showing off with wheel backbends, an ego-driven pose that can actually be bad for your body—men have a hard time doing them, but I would do them just to look cool. Now, I found my approach to yoga was evolving as well.

I was less concerned about how I looked doing a pose and was much more focused on how I *felt* doing the pose. I started learning less about how to do yoga and more about what yoga was. Lucky for me, my first teacher and still good friend, Colleen, was also wanting to go in a different direction with both her practice and her teaching. She wanted to sign up for a class on teaching "street yoga" and encouraged me to go with her. More than anything else I had done up to this point, this may have been what most prepared me for the yoga teaching I was to do in prison and beyond.

The instructors for street yoga opened my eyes to a world of teens in trouble, some of whom would clearly become adults in trouble. In this training, the teachers talked about the school-to-prison pipeline and how young people would fall into that cycle. I knew very little about it but could see the benefit "the power of the practice" (as these leaders called it) would have for at-risk youth—some of whom were homeless, others who were already trapped in the revolving door of the criminal justice system.

I learned about the work of yogi Bryan Kest, who, among other things, coined my favorite yoga phrase: "We bring our shit to yoga and we make yoga shit." By that he meant that we bring our judgments, self-doubts, and competiveness from our daily lives onto our yoga mat. Instead of releasing these attributes, many times our yoga practice increases our frustrations, self-doubts and competitiveness. When we fall out of a pose, rather than smiling, many times we get mad or frustrated that we can't do yoga. We have to be cautious that we're not strengthening the part of us that believes we're not good enough.

I saw it too often in the classes I was teaching at the health club and classes I attended at various other studios. Rather than accepting where others are in their journeys and their attempts at yoga, I saw judgment of other people's failures and clothes, and even their yoga mats. The point of using yoga is to let go of judgment and ego and just use it for release from ourselves and the darker side of human nature.

Yoga teaches that we are perfect the way we are: it does not try to change anyone; it should cultivate and nurture the qualities we already possess to be better people, not reinforce bad habits and thoughts. At a time when I very much needed it, I was finding release in yoga—I was letting go of old ways of looking at the world and adopting new ones.

As I was running classes, I stopped thinking of myself as the teacher. I wanted to instruct the participants in the poses, but when it came to the real value of yoga, I came to understand that the students have to teach themselves instead of being dependent on the teacher. It has been said that in the United States, we take two percent of yoga and make it the whole practice. We get the physical poses right and get everything else wrong.

In addition to my street yoga training, I started going to yoga retreats and workshops, as well as doing yoga outreach with several youth centers. Just before my sentencing, with very fortunate timing, I went to a power yoga workshop taught by one of the most respected yoga instructors in the world, Baron Baptiste. He had helped start a trend of sports teams doing yoga for strength and flexibility, and at one point in his career had been on the training staff of the Philadelphia Eagles football team.

Baptiste was one of my favorite yoga personalities because he was a leader not only in the athletic aspects of the practice, but in the meditative and psychological aspects of it as well. As a result of his workshop, I resolved to create a mantra for myself, to carry me through my sentencing and—if prison was to be my fate—through my incarceration.

Joy.
Surrender.
True self.

I didn't know what was going to happen in the next days and weeks, and I wanted to find joy in any way I could, under what I knew would be very different and difficult circumstances. I had to surrender to what was coming. I would have to stay true to myself no matter what happened: not become institutionalized, not give in to the baser aspects of human nature, which I suspected were thriving in the inmate culture.

I knew I was asking a lot of myself, but I knew I had yoga and the support of my friends to fall back on. I was in as good a spiritual place as I possibly could have been when, two-and-a-half years after entering a plea, I finally had a sentencing date: November 21, 2011. Even though I knew there was a chance that the sentence could be prison, I almost wanted to go and get it over with, if that was indeed what was coming. If I had started even the maximum sentence—twelve months—at the time I first pleaded guilty, I'd have been out by now and getting on with my life.

Chapter Four
Sentencing

*A judge's job is to judge others. I don't judge others,
because how we judge others is how we judge ourselves.
I'm tired of judging myself.*

At least intellectually, I knew that once I pleaded to a charge that could result in a prison sentence, I had to be prepared for spending time behind bars. All of our lawyers were making cases for the reasons why none of us deserved prison time. Many of my friends and family were trying to reassure me that there was no way I would actually go to prison. After all, they said, no one goes to a federal prison for a misdemeanor. Although I appreciated their optimism, I didn't know whether they were trying to convince themselves that I couldn't possibly be going away, or that they didn't fully understand the situation.

In the manner of awaiting the results of a biopsy, friends try to be supportive, offering assurance that the results will likely be benign. But they haven't been in the doctor's office for every appointment; they don't know what the patient knows. Although he can't be certain either until the results are in, he has a better notion or more-informed gut feeling than any outsider.

My case was complicated and the lawyers, all seasoned, top-notch counsel, dealt with the twists and turns as we, the very inexperienced defendants, tried to understand them. Warning flags indicated that things would not go our way. I tried to stay calm, doing my yoga and my meditations, and bracing myself for whatever may come, good or bad.

It is usual to ask friends, family, and colleagues for letters of support to try to demonstrate that the defendant is a good person and an asset to society, and why the judge should be lenient. The rules require the judge to read the letters, but who knows if he or she really does? In my case, we had nearly one hundred letters, far more than the norm. That is a lot of reading. We tried to arrange them in a logical order and to present a summary of them in the sentencing memorandum that we filed with the court. It would paint a picture of who Mike Huggins was as a person, broken down into the areas of my life: family, work, community engagement, and so forth.

People often say how interesting it would be to attend their own funerals, to hear the eulogies that would be given. Without having to die, the letters I received were an amazing tribute, and it was touching and heartwarming to read such warm words. It makes me wonder why we don't say those things to our friends before they die or go to prison.

Maybe it was more a measure of how well some people wrote than what they thought of me, but some whom I thought would write better letters had almost nothing to say. Others for whom I had low expectations wrote amazing letters. Some wrote things that surprised me with a depth of feeling and a level of respect I never knew they had for me; I was touched, and at times moved to tears by the letters. Some friends created a new level of relationship, which continued into my incarceration and out the other side.

I've always been a worrier and through this entire process tried to sort out my own negative notions from what I knew. We thought we had made a good case as to why I shouldn't go to prison at all, let alone be dragged away that day. But after we had an evidentiary hearing in June 2011, and then didn't hear from the judge until shortly before the November sentencing—when he issued a seventy-page opinion—I had little doubt I was going to prison.

The Thursday before sentencing, my yoga friends, including Colleen, gathered with me at a restaurant for what we knew might be a last supper. In spite of the seriousness of my situation, there was little mention of what was to come, and I felt little sadness. A big part of yoga is being in the moment. There was no "woe is me" attitude or cursing my fate. There were no tears but just a fun time with good friends. While there was no denying what might happen on Monday, more than anyone there, I wanted to concentrate on the positive, to allow this warm feeling of friendship to stay with me through whatever lay ahead.

My family all wanted to come to the sentencing, but one of my nephews got married in Washington, DC, on the Saturday prior to my court appearance, and it would have been difficult for many of them to make that pivot and be in court in Philadelphia, first thing Monday morning.

I didn't want my parents there anyway. If things went badly, I feared it would be too hard on them. I was thinking: best case, I am not doing jail time at all; most likely outcome, I am going, but will self-report later, so I'll have time to get my affairs in order and say my good-byes; worst case, if I'm hauled away in irons, I don't want them to see that. Their presence was either not necessary or not a good thing.

I skipped the wedding. With so much on my mind and not being in the mood to party, I wasn't sure I should be there. So many people in the family were aware of my situation that I also didn't want my presence to overshadow the happy day, with people expressing their condolences to me.

The night before my sentencing, the house was quiet. There seemed little doubt that prison was in my future. The only question was whether it would come tomorrow or in a few weeks. I took some time to digest the possibility that my sentence could very well start in the morning. I meditated with a rum and Coke in my hands.

— — —

Early Monday morning, Jenny, my daughters, and a few close friends went with me to court. Although Jenny and I were separated, she was very supportive through this process, and it certainly would look good to the judge to show my loving family standing behind me. We stopped at the Dunkin' Donuts across the street from the federal courthouse in downtown Philadelphia. Although I tried to be as upbeat and optimistic as possible, I cherished that cup of coffee as I harbored a strong suspicion that this could be my last decent coffee for a long time. I didn't eat anything. My stomach was too tight for that. Everyone tried to smile, but there was a worried bit of gallows humor to our brief breakfast.

The judge was brutal. From his written opinion, I was not expecting him to go easy, but the harshness of his tone and words surprised everyone. If I had been charged and convicted of the despicable things to which the judge was now referring, I would have spent my last dime and risked a hundred years in prison to prove my innocence.

He was sentencing us as if we had been convicted of the charges that had never been brought against us.

However, rather than get angry or frustrated, I went inward and started meditating with a focus on being aware of all that was happening: from the judge's words, the layout of the court room, the stacks of legal binders in front of the prosecutor, the stenographer, news reporters, friends, and my family—especially my family. To this day, I can remember all the sights, sounds, and emotions as if it happened yesterday. Clearly the judge's words were meant to be personal, yet somehow I didn't take it personally. There was a script in play here where an outcome seemed preordained, and yet I found myself going back to the Four Agreements—most notably, not taking things personally.

I was the first to stand in front of the judge. He treated me as though I was the kingpin of some wretched criminal conspiracy and acted as though it was his responsibility to make an example of me. I was willing to apologize for management mistakes, but I wasn't going to lie and take responsibility for things I didn't know about or do. Instead, I made myself ready for what seemed like a foregone decision.

Joy. Surrender. True self.

I couldn't change what had led to this moment—not the mistakes at Synthes, not my plea, not the judge's approach. I couldn't change what was coming next. There was only this moment. For good or bad, this was the moment. I had to live in it and accept it.

And time stood still. I have heard people describe car accidents. Years later, they were able to vividly recall every detail of the moment when they were sure they would die. The colors in the shattering glass, the screams of those around them. It was as though everyone in the courtroom was frozen and I could study everything. The way the judge was glaring at me. The pattern of the floor tiles. My lawyer's breathing. I could still hear distinctly every word the judge was saying, but it was also far away—like the voice from a television in the next room that somehow wasn't really directed at me. I was totally present, and yet not there. It was a combination of an out-of-body experience and one where I was very much grounded. It was one of the richest moments of my life, with vivid sounds, images, and smells. Even at the time, it struck me as surreal that this amazing experience was also happening in the worst moment of my life.

As the highest-ranking officer, I got the longest sentence: nine months. And he ordered me taken away immediately. After the briefest of hugs with Jenny and each of my daughters, I was handcuffed in front of my sobbing family and friends and led out a side door of the courtroom. I was too stunned to cry or express much emotion at all.

— — —

The sentencing hearing was relatively brief. It started at 8:00, and by 9:30 I was in a holding cell in the courthouse. The guards took all of my personal items and also my suit jacket, belt, tie, and shoelaces—suicide precautions, I guess. I was fingerprinted, photographed, and processed, and then placed in another holding cell, about 20-by-20, with a bench and an old metal, indestructible toilet.

I was glad I had some time by myself to try to settle my thoughts. For all of everyone's optimism, I suspected this might happen. Now I had to come to terms with it. Alone in the cell I repeated my mantra and reminded myself that whatever happened next, this was going to be a time of profound change and, hopefully, growth.

It still seemed hard to fathom. One minute I was standing in a courtroom in a suit, and less than two hours later, I was behind bars, stripped of anything potentially lethal. There would be lots of time not just in this cell, but in the many days to come, to try to make sense of this situation that was, on many levels, senseless.

Joy. Surrender. True self.

I didn't know what would happen next and really hadn't taken time to develop a self-defense strategy for being in prison. I didn't know if I would need one, but I had given little thought to what might happen once I was behind bars. I'd just try to blend in, at least until I had a better idea of the lay of the land.

Although none of the marshals informed me of anything, I had the distinct impression that the people processing me weren't ready for a new prisoner coming from the courthouse that early in the morning.

I'd never had a traffic ticket. I had never been arrested—even through this whole process, I had not been arrested. I was arraigned and had preliminary court appearances, but at no point had I entered the system. This seemed to be a little confusing for the people who were supposed to process me. They seemed more used to people coming from the Federal Detention Center to court, not headed in the other direction.

The system moves very slowly and isn't prepared to handle surprises. Most prisoners get to self-report, or they arrive from being arrested and are processed in some other way. I was some sort of an anomaly. Eventually other prisoners were let into my cell. Most were being brought to testify in a trial or were being taken to a bail hearing. All of the other detainees were already in the system, and I felt out of place as the only one not in a prison jumpsuit. I got curious looks from each of the prisoners as they were brought in. After I had been there a while, I had to go to the bathroom but wasn't sure how to do it. What was the protocol for taking a piss with strangers a few feet away? And it wasn't like a trough urinal in a stadium—just an open toilet with no partitions or screens around it.

After another four or five hours—it was hard to track time with no watch and no clock, under such unfamiliar circumstances—we were shackled and taken like a chain gang, through an underground tunnel to the basement of the FDC. There I was formally transferred from the custody of the U.S. Marshals to the custody of the federal Bureau of Prison (BOP) authorities.

Although the Marshals had taken my fingerprints, mugshot, and filled out intake forms, instead of giving this information over to the BOP, the BOP did all of the same things in a slightly different way.

The processing in and out of different institutions was to be repeated so many times that it eventually became just another annoying routine. It might have made sense if they were checking to make sure I was the same man who had been turned over, but no one seemed to be comparing the fingerprints or photographs. As someone who tried to make manufacturing work more economically, seeing this incredible, wasteful inefficiency frustrated my business mind and my inner taxpayer in so many ways. But it was what it was. I was where

I was. I could either go with the flow or drive myself crazy trying to understand or contradict it.

The people processing me into the FDC asked for my number. I had been told it once, but I certainly didn't have it memorized. The guard seemed disproportionately angry that I didn't know it and made it clear I shouldn't forget it again. From now on I was not Michael Huggins; I was 60419066.

The prisoners who were just in court for the day went right back into their cells. I was put into another holding cell with a few others who were still in civilian clothes. They told us to strip and took our clothes and boxed them up to be shipped home. We were issued prison jumpsuits. I was officially an inmate.

After more waiting, I was given a stale bologna sandwich—imitation bologna, if there is such a thing, on stale bread, and some orange sugar water to drink—a bad imitation of Kool-Aid, I guess. As bad as it was, I was glad I ate it, because it turned out to be all I'd be given all day.

Over the course of hours, the cell filled up. The guards brought in prisoners from other prisons or cells who were also new to the FDC, until at one point we had about three hours with just three of us. We talked and got to know each other a bit. It felt good to have people to talk to who shared my plight. Just small talk, really. There seemed to be an unspoken code to not discuss our crimes. Eventually someone came to take us to our cells. My long-awaited, inescapable prison sentence was about to begin.

Chapter Five
A Cell in the Cradle of Liberty

Good luck? Bad luck?
Luck is simply a perspective.
Happiness is determined by the self, not by events.

I was put on the elevator and told to face the back wall. It seemed odd to not be able to see where the elevator was going.

It was going to take a while to stop taking things personally, to realize that so much of what at first seemed planned inhumanity was really more just a profoundly callous bureaucracy at work. It has been said that the opposite of love isn't hate; it's indifference. The guards didn't hate me, they just didn't care.

Why should it bother me so much? Why did it matter which way I faced in an elevator? Just to watch the numbers light up? Since I didn't know which floor was mine and someone was going to tell me where to get off, why did it bug me not to face the door? Small inconveniences like facing the back of the elevator reminded me that my life and my choices were not my own for the foreseeable future. I had never been in a prison before, not even to visit anyone. I didn't associate with the kind of people who went to jail. I had no real concept of what to expect when the elevator doors opened and I was allowed to turn around.

The ride to the seventh floor seemed to take forever, but also not long enough. I wanted time to brace myself for what came next. All I knew about prisons came from watching movies and TV shows, and they certainly didn't show them as any place I'd want to go or be able to fit in. But any worrying I could do wasn't going to change whatever awaited me when I exited the elevator.

I reminded myself that I did have a choice. I could choose to give in to the panic I felt rising in me every few minutes, or I could choose to maintain my breathing and stay focused. Try to relax in this extremely uncomfortable situation. And surprisingly, I was able to keep relatively calm: Joy. Surrender. True self.

It was now 8:30 at night. With the speed I was soon to discover was the norm in the prison system, it had taken almost eleven hours to get me across the street and upstairs. It might have been a five-minute walk, had I gone directly over with no processing.

I was released into a common area with tables and chairs attached to the floor. There were small, sturdy metal doors regularly spaced around the outer edges. Everything about the surroundings was as drab as possible. It was as though they had given an interior designer the order to find the dullest colors and materials for everything—the tables, chairs, walls, cell doors, and even the uniforms. They were not the orange coveralls common in TV shows or the cliché black and white stripes, but just drab green one-piece jumpsuits, presumably designed to be as ill-fitting as they were on almost everyone, making even the men wearing them look monotonous, in spite of their otherwise very different looks. All ages and races seemed to be represented among my fellow inmates, but most fell into two types: guys who had just answered a casting call for "street thug," and guys who could have starred in a remake of *The Godfather.*

Men sat watching a television set that had been wheeled into the area, but they watched in silence—each man had earphones plugging his ears and was listening to the audio through his own small radio. There were a few men scattered around the periphery, reading. I was trying to take this all in. There was a lot of noise. Many men had the volume up so high on their earbuds that the indistinct noise could be heard twenty feet away. There were numerous conversations going on around the room, and a mix of sounds echoed off the metal railings and cell doors, creating a cacophony that was stressing my already frayed nerves.

Given my spork and indestructible plastic cup, I had been admonished not to lose them because they would not be replaced. I had my miniscule amounts of toothpaste and soap and other essentials that were supposed to suffice until I could get my actual rations of these things. The toothbrush I got was a finger brush. Sort of a condom for a fingertip, with bristles. Better than nothing, I guess.

It was a lot to try to absorb all at once. Although I was afraid, I wasn't terrified, and I also wasn't really sure what, if anything, I should be afraid of. For all of the craziness of the situation, I wasn't sure there was anything life threatening to fear. I wondered if there was enough supervision by guards and what might happen before they intervened. Or did their indifference extend to letting the prisoners sort things out for themselves?

There is anxiety on the first day of anything new—school, job, house—but prison was at a much higher level. This was a much more unfamiliar situation and carried potentially fatal or other serious consequences for a misstep.

— — —

Through the common area, I was led to my cell. On the bottom bunk was an African American man who seemed a bit startled by my arrival. I barely had time to take a look at him and my new home when the door was closed and locked behind me. I was sealed in a very small, dimly lit room with a complete stranger, knowing nothing about him or his crime.

I had not been given any orientation or explanation of what was going on, nor an introduction to my new roommate. Since he was in the bottom bunk, I clearly was supposed to take the top bunk. There was a small metal ladder up, but clearly it was going to take some care to get up and down without kicking or otherwise disturbing the man below.

With my admission to this cell, I was to notice a pattern that would repeat each time I was assigned to a cell or prison cubicle: a mild resentment on the part of the current occupants. Nothing personal, but that feeling you'd get as the plane doors are about to close and you're thinking that the seat next to you will remain empty for the entire flight, then at the last minute someone fills it. It's nothing against that person, but there is a twinge of animosity against someone who has taken a big chunk of my personal space, if only temporarily. Of course, in a prison situation, that person could be in my space for days or months, so the resentment is commensurately higher.

Dwayne, my cellie, was not particularly friendly or unfriendly. His familiarity with the system made it clear this was not his first time in the joint, and I had already deduced it was best not to ask what anyone was in for. He treated me decently. Here he was, a black guy from the streets of Philly, but during our brief time as roomies, somehow we found a good bit to talk about. People are people. At this juncture, Dwayne had far more useful knowledge than I did, so although I didn't exactly want his friendship, I did want his help.

I found that certain people were somewhat helpful because it was in their best interest to be. For instance, Dwayne told me about the stand-up count that happened at 9 o'clock. If the count was messed up, it would have to be done again, which could mean thirty minutes or more of standing for the recount or recounts. It was in Dwayne's best interest to tell me that I was to stand by the small slit window in the cell door so as the guards came by they could easily see both cellmates were present and accounted for. Another guard followed in the first guard's wake, doing an independent count. Then they'd compare numbers. If there was a discrepancy, we'd all have to stand there until it was reconciled.

Dwayne had a tiny radio that he played all day and night. The only radios sold through the commissary were designed only to be used with headphones, but some of the men had figured out how to modify the headphones as mini-speakers. The sound quality was tinny and annoying, but amazingly loud given the miniscule size of the thing. I wasn't sure if it was against prison etiquette to ask him to turn it off, but I doubted I was going to get much sleep that first night anyway, as nervous and keyed up as I was. I had just a rough blanket that would provide little comfort.

I tried to use the (relative) quiet to mentally and emotionally adjust to my new situation. Once again I focused on my mantra and renewed my resolve to use this time to learn whatever lessons I could. If I have a really horrible experience at a restaurant, I can either be angry or just decide I have learned something: never to eat there again. I knew there would be many new experiences coming, and as I hoped never to repeat prison, I should take away whatever teachings awaited—good and bad. From what I had seen so far there would be a lot of bad. But when I would have those thoughts, I'd try to remind myself that in Eastern philosophy, things are neither good nor bad. They just are. Any label of "good" or "bad" is a judgment someone has placed on that thing or event.

During my purgatory years, I had done a deep dive into philosophy and spirituality and found that my life philosophy was tending toward the Eastern ways of looking at the world, Buddhist thought in particular. As I considered my fate, I thought of the old Taoist parable that asks, "Is it good luck or bad luck?"

There is a story of a Chinese farmer and his son. The only thing they own of any value is a horse that they use to plow their fields. One day the horse runs away. The neighbors come over and say to the farmer, "You have such bad luck." And he replies, "How do you know?"

The next day the horse returns. It is a mare in heat and it is trailing twenty wild stallions. The farmer and his son are able to corral the wild horses. Now they have twenty-one horses! They will be able to sell many of them and will be rich.

The neighbors come over and say to the farmer, "You have such good luck." And he replies, "How do you know?"

The next day the farmer's son is trying to break one of the stallions, gets thrown, and shatters his leg. He'll never walk again. He won't be able to work the farm.

The neighbors come over and say to the farmer, "You have such bad luck." And he replies, "How do you know?"

The next day the army comes through and is rounding up all of the young men in the village to fight in a war. Everyone knows most of those young men will not be coming back. They take all of the young men except the farmer's son, who can't walk.

The neighbors come over and say to the farmer, "You have such good luck." And he replies, "How do you know?"

When things happen, there is usually no way of knowing in the short term if those occurrences are good or bad.

What I took away from my current situation would in large part hinge on whether I thought of this as good luck or bad. And since I couldn't change the circumstances, I might as well resolve that this was a good thing and make the best of it. Listening to Dwayne's radio and trying to find a comfortable position on this horrible bunk made it difficult to see how, at the present moment.

The next morning my cellmate told me to hurry—breakfast was being served out in the common area. Little kindnesses like that which really didn't benefit Dwayne made me think he was an okay guy in spite of some of his quirks. I wanted to have the cereal provided; I was still hungry from the day before. As I looked around for a seat, I spotted Eddie, with whom I'd come up to the floor. He seemed like a safe enough bet and I went to sit with him. It felt good to at least have one somewhat familiar face to which I could say hello.

During the few weeks that we were together on the seventh floor, I continued to see Eddie and hung out with him periodically. Eventually a friend of his from another prison also showed up on our floor. It was weird how many people seemed to know each other. I knew no one in the system; I was the perennial new kid in school. How was there this vast world and network of people out there of which I was so completely unaware? I had read that over two million people in this country were behind bars—just less than one percent of the population. And millions more had done time and been released. How had I never crossed paths with them to know about this vast community?

One thing that made me particularly nervous about Dwayne was his using our cell as a phone booth. He and some friends—or perhaps business associates, although I certainly didn't want to ask what business was being conducted—had figured out that it was possible to talk through the toilet. He would ask me to leave the cell, so I never got a good look at what was going on, nor did I want to, but they would stack their plastic cups to make a tube about two and a half feet long. They would insert the tube into the toilet and talk to the people in the cell on the floor below. It was just one of the many surreal moments I would encounter as my life changed. Who would know to try this? How did they arrange call times with their buddies and know the right cells to use?

Dwayne had been in and out of prisons and other detention facilities much of his life and seemed surprised that I could know so little of a system he knew well enough to know how to work around it. He put his shock aside to answer the questions he could. He wasn't forthcoming about a lot of stuff, but if I asked he'd answer. He warned when I was about to cross some invisible line of prison etiquette that might have gotten me in trouble with a guard or another prisoner.

The prison authorities threw newbies into the deep end and expected them to swim. Dwayne may not have been the friendliest guy going, and was a little scary in some ways, but he was my only orientation to the FDC. I heard of guys whose cellmates had not been at all helpful and were left to fend for themselves or to seek out a mentor among the other prisoners, with mixed results.

Among other things, I had to learn the language of the incarcerated. The guards were usually referred to as COs (correctional officers) or simply as "cops." I started using phrases like "on the street" and "down a long time," and I had to learn how commissary worked.

I felt like Alice in Wonderland: I was in an alternate universe that exists underground that no one above ground knows much about. There were rules and customs here with which everyone seemed familiar except me.

Most of the guys had grown up in the system. They went from juvenile hall to county jail to state prison or the federal penitentiary. They moved from one level to the next, the way I had gone from kindergarten to elementary school to college to grad school. It would be like someone going to a PhD-level class if he had never learned the basic protocol of how school worked: how to get the teacher's attention, how to address the teacher, what homework was or how to do it. That's how I felt. I was clueless about everything from how to make a phone call to my family to: what is the etiquette for using the toilet when my cellmate is three feet away? There was never a class on this at Villanova or Wharton.

About 6:30 every morning, the cells opened one by one. Chow was fast. We got it and ate it quickly. Almost everyone went back to bed, but I knew there was slim chance of getting back to sleep, so I would often use this opportunity to practice walking meditation. I would try to do it out in the rec area if the weather was okay, but of course that meant doing laps of a very small area. Inside there was a bit more space, but also more obstacles and people to interrupt the flow during laps.

The rec area was a small outside "patio" about the right size for a half-court game of basketball, and there was a hoop and a ball, and since this was one of the few forms of recreation offered, games went on even on the coldest days as long as we weren't on lockdown. It was the only bit of sun and sky and fresh air that some of these men had experienced for months. I wasn't sure how long I could take this sort of confinement, but I had hoped that I would be leaving soon. ("Soon," with the relative speed of the BOP, I was to learn is still very slow.)

After breakfast, our cell doors would be left open until about 10 a.m., then we'd be locked down for an hour or so for a count and whatever maintenance needed to be done. Most of the work was done by women inmates, who occupied half of the building and, with the exception of serving meals, they held virtually all of the jobs. Few men served their full sentences at the FDC, but many women did long stretches there, so they could be trained to do the more skilled jobs, including electrical and plumbing around the place.

Then we again stood by the little window until the count was clean. After lunch we were free until about 3 p.m., then back in our cells until the 4:30 count. We'd be released for dinner and the door left open until after 9, when there'd be the final count and lights out.

Living in very close quarters with a complete stranger, especially one from whom there was no separation for twelve or so hours a day, was a challenge, to say the least. Our first little conflict came when, after about four days of no sleep at all due to his loud radio, I asked if it might be possible to turn it down. I had tried everything—wadding up toilet paper to use as ear plugs, wrapping my blanket around my head—anything to try to muffle the noise. His answer was that I snored so loud that he needed the music to drown out my snoring. That was sort of an impasse and apparently, I was just going to have to learn to deal with the radio.

When either Dwayne or I needed to use the toilet, the other guy would look away. When it wasn't lockdown and one of us was able to be in the common area, he left the room to give some privacy, and we'd each place a towel over the peep hole in the door so other people couldn't see in and would know not to walk in.

Like several other African Americans I was to encounter in prison, Dwayne was what I came to refer to as a born-again Muslim. He was embracing his new faith. Far be it from me to stop someone on their spiritual journey regardless of what that might be, especially if it didn't impinge on me in any way. But there was one way his chosen religion did. We had a little argument because he wanted me to pee sitting down.

"It's how we do it in my religion," he said.

I tried to tell him that his religion was his religion, and I preferred to stand to do my business. He wasn't happy about this. I had Muslim friends and coworkers on the outside, and this was the first I had ever heard of this. Of course, how often does anyone ask a coworker or friend about their bathroom habits?

It wasn't until I got out of prison that I finally had a chance to investigate this. Apparently it's true: devout Muslims think it's unclean to stand to urinate. Who knew?

Chapter Six
Learning to Suffer

Yoga is not about having fancy workout clothes or even a mat,
but about finding comfort in the present moment,
enjoying each breath, and becoming comfortable in your own skin.

The FDC itself was an interesting setup. I had been to Philadelphia's historical district hundreds of times and had never noticed it. It is so nondescript that after I got out, when I would tell people I had been in a federal detention facility one block from Independence Mall and three blocks from Independence Hall itself, they would say that was impossible—they would have noticed a prison there. When I went back, I realized there is almost nothing on the outside that would indicate that the high-rise building is actually a prison. It has narrow windows, but no major signage, and the barbed-wire-enclosed balconies are recessed in such a way that unless anyone knew to look really hard at them, they wouldn't notice that odd adornment that set it apart from any other office tower in the city.

There were four wings on eight floors of cells; some wings were for women, but most were for men. I heard there were close to a thousand people housed in this building. The entire top floor was reserved for the SHU. Pronounced "shoe," it was an acronym for Special Housing Unit, also known as "solitary" or "the hole." If an inmate caused too big a problem, that's where he went. Almost no privileges—they were very few in the general population of the FDC, but in the SHU there were none—and no contact with anyone, locked in a tiny cell twenty-three hours a day, meals slipped through a slot in the door the way animals at the zoo were fed. It was not a place I ever wanted to go or even see, and even hardened, experienced inmates seemed to want to avoid a trip to the SHU at all costs.

For most men, the FDC was transitional, but some of my fellow inmates said they thought that since I was in for such a short sentence, the BOP might not even bother moving me to a camp or any other prison—that I would be stuck in the FDC for my entire nine months. I just had to hope and pray that wasn't the case.

For my first week at the FDC, there was no staff on duty to create an account to be able to call or email—those services were on hiatus for Thanksgiving week. Staff were off work, offices were closed, and services weren't available. I eagerly awaited the day when I could reconnect with the outside world and be reassured it still existed.

There were four email terminals housed in a small room for inmate use. The room was open for limited hours, and there was always a line of a dozen or more men deep to get in and use them. There was no word processing program on these units—they weren't even full computers—just direct access to the BOP's own email system. I had to request that people be put on my email list, as I could not just contact anyone I wished. I paid by the minute to be online, and there was no way to compose messages offline to copy and paste them into an email. Not very convenient or efficient for someone like me who had a lot to say.

— — —

I soon learned that my next lesson in prison culture would test my intuition and ability to believe people, and leave me questioning my judgment. I noticed a man in the common room area reading interesting books. I asked about one and Philip began to lend me his books.

One of the first books of his that I read was to have more of a profound influence on me than just about any other book I read during my time in prison: *The Heart of the Buddha's Teaching*, by Thich Nhat Hanh. It was the right book at the right time for me. It has often been said that when the student is ready, the teacher will appear, and Thich Nhat Hanh was the teacher I needed at that moment. The book resonated across any religion, from Buddhism to Catholicism. It was about the common spirituality inherent in all religions and how those tenets could guide a good life and lead one to inner peace. Among the things that resonated with me from the book were Four Noble Truths:

1. There is suffering.
2. We should be aware of the nature of suffering, or how we create suffering for ourselves.
3. We can learn how to stop suffering.
4. The eightfold path shows us how to refrain from things that cause suffering.

The book also caused me to examine what suffering is. For some, a picnic on the beach is the ideal way to spend a day. For someone who is sensitive to the sun and can't handle the heat, it could be their worst day ever. It also had the same to say about joy: what is joy for one (again—a day at the beach) is hell for someone else. It is the dual nature of everything. Is the beach good or bad? Neither. It's just the beach. Anything else is just a value judgment we place on it.

Another important lesson I was to take from the book was the concept of interbeing: the idea of the connectedness of all people and all things. This is not a new concept, certainly, and has been expressed in many ways by poets and philosophers—the idea that no man is an island: what hurts anyone hurts me. I had already been reading about and considering the concept of nondualism, and this fit in quite closely with that. There is no difference between myself and anyone else. It is easy to see others as different: he is in prison, therefore he is different. But now I was in prison and no different than anyone else who was. We tend to see people as their differences: different gender, different skin color, different age, different sexual orientation, but there are no real differences—we all share the same DNA as human beings. And although I still didn't consider myself a new-age disciple, reading Thich Nhat Hanh had me understanding even more clearly that we are all one, and that any barriers between us are artificial and can be transcended to bring us together as one.

Although I was a long way from forming even the smallest inkling of a new future career for myself, I was already thinking about my responsibility (something Thich Nhat Hanh writes about) for making the world better. I found the book fulfilling and I devoured it, wanting to both read it quickly and savor the best parts, like a great meal.

Other gems of wisdom stuck with me and started me on my new path, including acknowledging our co-responsibility for each other. Young people harm themselves and others because life has no meaning for them. If we give them a reason to live and flourish, they will. I had been trying to take more responsibility for paying my rent on this planet as a member of the human race. Now I had time to reflect on how that might be possible. I saw it in the street yoga training, and was already seeing here at the FDC, the ways in which our society fails to teach people how to live—how to deal with anger, how to reconcile conflicts, how to breathe, smile, and transform situations.

I resolved to smile and nod to everyone I encountered: to acknowledge each person, if only in a small way. Someone I told about this thought I was crazy—that under the circumstances, to make eye contact with the wrong person was dangerous. Rather than putting myself at risk, I felt that by making even a small connection, I was less likely to get attacked by anyone. I was not threatening in any way, and if they could see me as human, that might be a good thing. I didn't want to try to project some hard-ass, street-tough persona that was definitely not me. It would likely come off as fake and would be seen through right away.

Strangely, after the initial fear passed in a day or two, I was not terribly afraid; but the entire time I was in the FDC, I never lost some element of fear. There was always some anxiety: not knowing the rules, both real and assumed, I was afraid I might cross some line with either a guard or another prisoner. There was always what I began to think of as "tense boredom"—the notion that something bad could happen at any time, although most of the time, pretty much nothing at all was happening.

In these bizarre surroundings, I thought about what Thich Nhat Hanh asked about finding life's purpose: did I have to have a purpose or was my purpose simply to be myself? I knew the spiritual journey on which I had embarked was my own. I would have to find my own way, find my own teachers, and teach myself.

I was eager to discuss the book with Philip. I thought he was someone I could relate to—someone also seeking his new path and truth and perhaps someone who could help guide me on my journey. New path aside, I wanted to see what other books Philip might have and be willing to lend me. None of my friends on the outside were able to send me books yet.

For many requirements, the BOP did the bare minimum: if two books were all that were required to have a library, they could check off that box on some form and not worry about it any longer. With the prison divided into wings, there was no way to have a central library with a wide selection of books available to all prisoners. In one corner of the common area were about twenty-five books, most of them in Spanish. I was so desperate for reading material that although I don't read Spanish, I might have gotten to the Spanish books had Philip not been there to provide reading material.

With little else to do but read—we were usually locked in our cells sixteen or more hours a day—I could consume a book in a day or three. Some days we'd only be allowed out for meals. We were expected to wolf down the food in minutes before being sent back to our cells. After a fight or incident, we'd be locked in our cells for hours or the rest of the day. If there had been an altercation, when we emerged from lockdown, the combatants were gone. We'd also be locked down during surprise drills for escapes, fires, and riots. Most times we'd have no idea why we had been confined to our cells.

That much time in my cell with a not very talkative roommate meant lots of time for books. Often, the only thing that slowed me from reading more was taking time to contemplate what I was learning from these readings. Philip and I were getting along quite well now, and we started eating some meals together. He did seem to be on his own spiritual path, and he had several other books of interest to me and was willing to loan them. Philip seemed happy to have found someone with whom to share his collection and exchange ideas.

He quoted poets, scholars, philosophers, and people I'd never heard of. He talked about the loving intimacy of Mark Nepo: "Asleep too long, we need to wake. Awake too long, we need to sleep."

Philip quoted Lao-Tzu: "When I let go of what I am, I become what I might be."

He became animated when talking about Rumi: "Yesterday I was clever, so I wanted to change the world. Today I am wise, so I am changing myself." Wow. Deep and impactful conversation in the least of expected places.

Until I started talking to him, he had kept very much to himself. He spoke to no one and no one spoke to him. I thought it was because he was a very spiritual guy and into communing with himself. He also wrote a lot, sitting in a corner, filling pages with his thoughts. After he saw me doing yoga, we began meditating together.

Then one day a menacing-looking white guy to whom I had barely spoken saw me alone and approached me. I had noticed the man because of his fierce demeanor and the entourage that he had collected. Word was he was in for a violent armed home-invasion robbery. He said to me, "That guy you're eating with is a child molester. You seem like an okay guy, and if there is trouble with him, you don't want to be part of it." He didn't make it sound like he was threatening me at all, but seemed to be giving me a legitimate warning. Like a stranger might say as he saw someone leaving a hotel, "You may want to take an umbrella, it's starting to rain."

It was just another part of the weird and enforced hierarchy in prison: child molesters were the lowest of the low, and everyone was better off keeping their distance from them. Word was this guy had taken vacations to foreign countries for prearranged sex with minors. I knew such things existed, but those things were so far removed from my world it was jarring to have that world show up at my lunch table. I stopped eating with Philip. Whether or not the story of his crimes was true, it was not worth risking the wrath of the home invasion guy and his posse. Or anyone else.

I had heard that child molesters and sexual predators were on the bottom of the food chain in prison. They often had to be kept in protective seclusion to prevent them from being harmed by other inmates. At the FDC, there was no separation between the men who were bound for maximum-security penitentiaries and those headed for minimum security, and no segregation based on the nature of anyone's crime.

Most inmates didn't talk or ask about other people's offenses, but if someone was curious enough, he could ask a friend on the outside to Google the accused. When I got out, Philip was the one person I did want to research; I had to try to reconcile the man I thought I knew with the pervert the news stories said he was. The stuff I read online was appalling. But I knew that if anyone Googled me, it would sound bad as well. I was never able to defend myself in print, so anyone who read about me would think the worst. Not as bad as Philip, certainly, but not good at all.

Some of Dwayne's cohorts who would come into the cell to use the "phone" were scary. They'd eye me with something close to malice. But soon Dwayne would calm them down with, "Mike's an okay guy." That seemed to soften their glares. Dwayne seemed to be one of the most popular guys on the wing and knew lots of people. He eventually began to express an interest in learning some things I knew about business, investments, and other religions or philosophies, and I was glad to repay the education he had given me when I first arrived.

Most of the guys on my wing were African American, and I got along okay with most of them. The majority of the white guys seemed like Mafia types whom I had zero interest in getting to know. There was one of the Mafia guys in particular to whom I took an almost instant dislike, due to his arrogance and his seeming need to have a small posse around him. I didn't need finely honed street smarts to know whom to avoid. In such a confined place, it was hard to completely avoid anyone, but I did try to give him, and most of the Mafia guys' devotees, a wide berth.

Occasionally the tension of our circumstances got the better of some men, and angry words became a shove or a punch. The guards were usually quick to intervene, for which I was grateful. If I somehow ran afoul of someone, I hoped help would be coming soon; I didn't want to be in the middle of a prison riot.

Whether these fights manifested on the spot because someone did something like cutting in line, or were due to a grudge carried in from the street, most of the time I didn't know—nor did I want to. Some of these men really scared me. And it wasn't an unwarranted fear. Some had already killed people. Others were going away for life and they knew it, so what was another murder or two tacked on to a sentence that would extend for centuries?

After the staff finally returned from their long holiday break, I was able to have access to the phones. They were pay phones, but instead of coins, we had to enter our access numbers to make a call. The phones were only available four or five hours per day—less if we were kept on lockdown. As soon as the phones were opened up, lines would form. Each call was limited to ten minutes. It was a challenge to make calls with so little time and so little privacy. I could get back in line when my time was up, but each person only had three hundred minutes a month—ten minutes a day is not a lot of time to stay connected.

One good thing the lines for the phones provided was a chance for interaction with some other people. It was awkward to just start random conversations, but while waiting in the phone queue, it was hard not to talk to someone in such close proximity. Often they were brief conversations, just a phrase or sentence—"How ya doing?"— but by this point I was getting a little starved for human interaction and welcomed those chats. I can't imagine how anyone survived solitary with no human connection. I had tried talking to people at meals, but with mixed results—and after the experience with Philip, I didn't want to become anyone's steady dining companion until I at least knew something about them.

In line I'd sometimes get asked, "When did you get in?" I looked like enough of a newbie that most guys did seem to think I was new, not just to the floor, but to any prison.

— — —

As soon as I could, I called Larry for some word about Bob. As I expected, it wasn't good. In addition to losing my brother, I felt bad that I couldn't be there for my daughters. They had never lost a close relative before, and I hated not being able to comfort them and myself by hugging them as they suffered this loss. I asked Larry to be there for them.

Not feeling comfortable confiding in anyone at the FDC, I started practicing walking meditation to calm myself. There was no gym or gym equipment, and I had noticed men doing whatever exercises they could: push-ups, modified chin-ups on their doors, press-ups on the tables.

I started doing more yoga, still of a conservative kind—nothing too odd or flashy. One day I was doing tree pose—standing on one leg, arms extended toward the ceiling when I noticed a few guys watching. When I returned my foot to the floor, one of the men asked, "Is that some sort of martial art? Like karate?"

"It's yoga," I replied.

"Really? That looks like a pretty good workout. Can you show me a couple moves?"

Soon more men were asking me to show them. As these informal classes grew, I asked if we might be able to use the little cinderblock room that was off the common area. I got another lesson in the rules of prison: the answer was no and yes. Some guards could see the benefit of yoga and happily let us use the room, welcoming the opportunity to let the prisoners unwind and exercise in this way; some of the guards were clearly indifferent to what the prisoners did as long as they weren't killing each other, so would open the room. Other COs wouldn't let us use the room and seemed upset that other cops had broken the regulations and let us in.

For these classes we had no mats, no blocks, no fancy yoga clothes. But rather than detract from these classes, those deficiencies made these sessions more impactful than any I had done in an expensive yoga studio with all of the right equipment. It was yoga distilled to its purest form. I knew many of the yoga poses would be inappropriate for a prison audience. I didn't want to do anything that would put the men in positions that might be embarrassing. I definitely didn't want to expose them or myself to ridicule. The windows into the cinderblock room meant anyone who cared to look could observe us. Poses such as downward dog, that has one's butt sticking up, and happy baby, that spreads the legs, seemed wrong for this setting.

One thing I noticed is that in prison no one talks about prison rape. On the outside, people joke about "dropping the soap," but here that thought was too close to home to ever be expressed. I never heard or saw any incidents, but it I certainly didn't want to turn off any potential yoga devotees by poses that might lead to comments.

I had learned a few things about working with special classes from the street yoga training, but many of the other techniques I figured out on my own. For one thing, I wanted to stick to English for all of the terms instead of Sanskrit, which is traditionally used. It was more likely that the guys would get it if I referred to something as tree pose instead of a *vriksasana* or a standing asana.

One of the things I liked about Colleen's style right from the start was that it was more invitational rather than dogmatic. These prisoners had failed at too many things in life, and it was important that they not feel as though they had failed at yoga. I had been to so many classes in so many different places in my decade of practicing that I had experienced many different styles. Some instructors came off like drill instructors barking instructions: "Raise your left leg! Higher! Get it up there!"

My friend Bruce and I once took an Ashtanga class together during one of our trips to Boston, from which we were dismissed.

First the instructor singled Bruce out and said, "You're done!"

"What do you mean 'done'?" Bruce asked.

"If you can't do the poses properly, get out!"

I thought it was funny, but when I failed a few poses later, I was also expelled from class: the instructor tapped me on the shoulder and said the same curt, "You're done!" Bruce never let me forget this. In retrospect it was hilarious, but it so turned him off to yoga that he never tried it again. Bruce and I still joke about him being a yoga dropout, but that is not how I wanted these men to feel in the FDC.

For the classes I was now teaching, it was important to make them approachable: "If it feels comfortable now to raise your left leg, go ahead and raise it. If that doesn't work for you, it's okay to leave it on the floor." Many had never done anything like this, weren't very flexible, or had other issues, so I wanted it to seem easy.

As soon as I could get on the email system, I sent a message to Jenny and Colleen. They were my conduits to the outside world and would forward my emails to a large (and soon to be growing) list of people who wanted to stay in touch. I was grateful to know that so many people cared about me and were eager for news of my well-being.

Dear Friends:

I hope this note finds you well.

I apologize for not being able to write to you, but there continues to be limited email access (can only have 10 people on email list). The visitation approval process continues to be chaotic as there hasn't been a counselor here in 9 days (he must approve the requests). Such is life in the slammer.

As someone who likes things organized and efficient, it has been a challenge to relax and not get overly frustrated.

Now into my 4th week and struggling with the slow passage of time. While continuing to focus on making each day the best I can, it's hard not to reflect on how much time I have left. 9 months seems like eternity. Yet compared to others here, 9 months is nothing. Most inmates are facing long periods of incarceration. I met a guy who has already served 25 years of a life sentence.

The good news is that I'm finding my way... I even did my first trade with an inmate... a pair of cheap earphones for food.

At the commissary, I was able to buy peanut butter and crackers, hot sauce, tea, shaving cream, disposable blades, toothpaste, toothbrush, shampoo, and deodorant. This may seem trivial but makes a huge difference in the quality of life. I used to take for granted brushing my teeth or shaving but now I really enjoy these mundane tasks. I only shave every other day so I can make the blades last longer.

I know my situation is unique, but I encourage you to try to slow down a bit and take the time to appreciate the little things in life. Try to see yourself moving in slow motion as you can see/experience every detail.

I continue to meet people through yoga. Class consists of several Muslims, Latinos, and Mafia types, and it's been a challenge to instruct the different personalities, age, and physical differences, but I think they all enjoy it and seem to understand the power of breathing.

Class is held in a small cement room with no mats or blocks, and inmates won't take off their socks. However, I have found this practice to be among the deepest I have ever experienced. After class all the anxiety and fear seem to disappear.

Where I had felt despair, I feel hope. Where I had felt lonely, I feel surrounded by loving support. Where I had felt sorry for myself, I feel empowered. Where I had felt this as a waste of precious life I feel that this experience will strengthen my calling when I'm "back on the streets."

A special thanks to Jenny, who has been my lifeline and who continues to carry the heavy burden without a complaint or without fanfare. She has been simply unbelievable.

Also thanks to all of you for your love and support. Words cannot describe what this means to me.

Love & gratitude,
Mike

One of those I had befriended through yoga was William. I had seen him quietly sketching in a pad. He was a tall black man, about twenty-one years old. One day as I was practicing some of my yoga poses, he approached me and asked me about what I was doing. He asked me if yoga could help him get six-pack abs. I answered that yoga could be very good for the core, and although I couldn't promise him a six-pack, I was willing to start training him.

He really took to it and had a natural ability and agility: the ease with which he adopted poses that had taken me months or years to master made him an awesome student. Before long we were working on what I considered the more important part of yoga—the mindful aspect.

Once he knew me well enough to trust me, he shared some of his story—a troubled upbringing in a bad neighborhood; it was a background out of a TV cop show or *60 Minutes* segment, not the sort of thing I ever expected to hear firsthand. Rumor had it that he had been involved in a drug deal that went bad and someone ended up dead. He and several of his accomplices were now scattered among the floors in this building awaiting trial. William seemed very remorseful that he had been a part of anything so wrong, although he never told me exactly what he was being tried for or what his part in any crime may have been.

He also shared his sketchbook with me. The output of his raw, untrained hand, using the very limited supply of pencils and pens available from the commissary was incredible. Amazing, innovative designs for clothing that seemed even more incongruous given the setting in which he was sketching them. He said he dreamed of going into fashion design someday, but wasn't sure how that could ever happen, especially now.

William seemed to have a good deal of cred on the wing and started bringing others into my makeshift yoga and mindfulness classes. Thanks to his recruiting, I'd sometimes have eight or ten guys in class.

The energy in that small room was so much more amazing than anything I had ever experienced under "ideal" yoga studio conditions.

It was sad to see this young man, clearly intelligent and thoughtful in spite of so little formal education, and yet so talented, embarking on what would apparently be a wasted life in prison.

I was far from a bleeding heart liberal, feeling much more at home with the white-collar crowd most of my life, but it was hard to see someone in such a horrible place, swept there by bad circumstances. I tried to think of what I could do to help him. It was hard not to wonder how different things could have been had he been born in a different neighborhood, with the opportunity to make different life choices.

Not knowing how long either he or I would be on the same wing, I wanted to do what I could to provide him with some tools to cope with what could be a long time—perhaps even a lifetime—behind bars. I could only hope some of the mindfulness techniques I shared with him helped in some small way.

Chapter Seven
Cheesesteaks and Support Bras

Let go of your bitterness.
You'll no longer define your life by how you've been hurt.
Define your life by compassion and understanding.

Still reluctant to make close friends, I was now making more acquaintances, and it was nice to have people with whom to converse. Now that I was no longer completely new and was not just soaking up information, I was able to share my own knowledge and skills with others.

In addition to yoga and some workout tips, the other topics about which many seemed eager to learn were the stock market and the legal system. It was something I was to see time and time again in the FDC and later in Lewisburg: the great thirst for knowledge regardless of socioeconomic class or formal education. Many guys would see someone who knew something they didn't, and they wanted to learn all they could from that person. Some of the white-collar guys were dismissive of those requests, but I not only didn't mind, I enjoyed it.

I thought most of the people I would meet in prison would deny the charges against them and claim they were framed or railroaded, but to my surprise, most of the guys were upfront about what they did. Many did complain about what a raw deal they got, their unfair sentences and the bad public defenders they had, but not everyone claimed innocence, although there were jokes that no one in the place was guilty.

Most of the guys said I was lucky to be going to a federal prison, agreeing that any federal pen was a hundred times better than a state prison. It was interesting to hear the men compare the pluses and minuses of the Pennsylvania state prisons to those of New Jersey or New York, as friends from my former life would compare vacationing in Ireland versus vacationing in Aruba.

Then came the inevitable speculation as to what would happen to me. Some who heard my story would say, "You're going to a camp because you shouldn't be in the pen anyway." Others, with just as much certainty and knowledge of the system said, "No, you're too short time, it's not worth them to do the paperwork to transfer you. I'm sure you'll do your full sentence here." As the days became weeks and the weeks became a month, it looked more and more likely.

I adapted as my situation changed, just as at a picnic I might eat that hot dog with a little dirt on it—something I would never do at home. What I considered edible or tolerable for food was changing rapidly in the FDC.

Not knowing whom to trust was more difficult than dealing with the lack of creature comforts and decent food. I would find myself liking someone but wondering what they were in for, and had to ask myself if I could trust them—they were in prison, after all. But then, so was I. I was wary about sharing too much information. I was a bit paranoid when someone was too nice; I'd wonder what he wanted from me. There are many, many people there I wouldn't trust at all. It was hard to know whom to believe or what the truth was. Especially after the experience with Philip, I tried to be cautious of forming relationships. However, one of our basic human needs is connection with our fellow man, so despite the circumstances, I tried my best to see the good in everyone.

Sometimes after I had divulged too much, I would then spend the long nights over-analyzing everything. After giving out my phone number or home address to a few people, I questioned the wisdom of doing this. There were a lot of dangerous men in there. Logic told me that I shouldn't share too much, and I struggled with how much to trust people who were felons. I'd always been an open and honest person, and it was hard to keep my barriers up.

— — —

With no place for personal space, I would seek refuge by retreating to my bunk and look out the sliver of a window. From my top bunk, I had a limited view of the sky and the world, but at least it was a view. Some of the cells, especially on the lower floors, had a view of essentially nothing.

One corner of a park could be seen through my window, though I wasn't sure if it extended beyond my line of sight for another ten feet or another ten blocks. I didn't know this part of Philadelphia well enough to know what park it was. Lying on my bunk, I would watch people coming and going from the grounds. As cold as it was, there weren't a lot of people hanging out there—perhaps in the summer, people would bring their lunches to eat on the benches that were within my limited view. Now anyone pausing on the benches stayed only briefly. I could also see part of a carousel, but it appeared to be shuttered for the winter. Just that little glimpse of normal people living normal lives in that park gave me an anchor in the real world, and for that I was grateful.

On the outside area I could stand on a chair and look out over a small slice of the Philadelphia skyline—as limited as my view of the outside world was, I enjoyed doing this to not feel quite so caged. One day I noticed the top of the PSFS building where my brother Bob had worked; I had visited him in his office. The building was one of the first skyscrapers in Philadelphia and is on the register of historic places. No longer an office building, it had been converted into a hotel in around 2000. From prison, it seemed odd to look up at that bastion of normal life and know I wasn't free to go there now. Suddenly I wanted to visit an office building which I hadn't been in for years and where Bob no longer worked. I wondered if, when Bob was still working there, he had ever looked down from his office and knew there was a prison in his line of sight. I wondered if he ever gave a thought to the unfortunate men and women locked up in the innocent-looking building a few blocks away.

I wondered a lot of things about Bob, but especially wondered if I would ever get to ask him anything ever again—whether about mundane details of his office or more major moments of his life.

Thinking and worrying seemed to go hand in hand. Logically, worrying solves nothing. Working out a constructive solution was one thing, but when I wasn't in a position to change things—where I'd be going next or whether Bob would live much longer—what was the point in worrying about it? I wanted to help the men in these yoga classes calm their inner voices, and I had found great success by focusing on body awareness. However, when dealing with so many new experiences and sensations, I would sometimes find it hard to practice what I was preaching.

There is a saying in yoga that people spend too much time in their heads and not enough in their bodies. An essential part of class was asking people to check in with their bodies. "How does your back feel? What tensions are you holding? What sensations are you feeling?" Focusing attention on sensations in the body can help relax the mind by allowing tensions to be released through the physical body and not be stored as pent-up frustrations or anger.

I desired a visit with my family to get some word about Bob, which might quell some of that anxiety, but I had just missed the last visitation for my wing due to Thanksgiving. Just as my wing's visitation day came up again, I was transferred from the seventh floor to the fourth. I found out I had just missed visitation for my new floor and would have to wait until the following week before I could have a visitor. Between the holiday and this frustrating turn of events, this would make almost three weeks inside without a visitor.

My family had been given incorrect instructions as to where to send money to put into my commissary account. This was a common problem, one that Piper Kerman wrote about in her book *Orange is the New Black*. After I got out, I read her book and found it strangely reassuring to find that so many of the "abnormalities" I encountered were apparently normal in the federal prison system—or at least Kerman and I ran into many of the same issues and challenges. Bad instructions were routine. There was always conflicting information, so it was hard to know whose instructions to follow. Each administrator had a different answer, and then some helpful (or not) inmate would say, "No, the way it really works is…"

Just when I finally had funds in my account and was about to have my commissary day to buy some necessities, I had been transferred—and, as with visitation, I had just missed commissary on the old floor and the new one.

When I stopped feeling sorry for myself, I'd try to remember there was no such thing as good luck or bad luck, just things that happened to us. I guess I could learn to do without the extras for another week or two.

Joy. Surrender. True self.

— — —

When I got transferred downstairs, I immediately noted that someone had stolen the mattress from my bunk. When I pointed out the lack of mattress to the guards, with their typical indifference they shrugged as though to say, "So?" I always said yoga was learning to accept an uncomfortable position. This was definitely challenging that mantra. I got no sleep, as I tried to find a way to place my body on bare metal with some degree of comfort. I would never look at homeless people sleeping on concrete the same ever again.

Even on a good night in the FDC, sleep was hard to come by, but on nights like this it was impossible, and I had too much time to consider my predicament. In my short experience in the prison system, I had already seen too many men who had fallen into that quicksand of despair and now not only couldn't save themselves but were also too far gone for anyone else to help them.

It wasn't as though I never gave into doubts and pondered, "How the hell did this happen to me?" But when I taught yoga, I would remind the class that if thoughts appeared, to just let them flow through and flow out. It is easy to say to someone, "Clear your mind," but it is much harder to do, especially if the person had no experience with meditation. It's not always possible for one to keep their mind blank, but anyone can learn to let go of thoughts instead of latching onto them, gnawing on them the way so many people do, with negative notions and fears. The other thing that I was to encounter to shake my worldview was to meet men who were almost grateful to be in prison. Their lives had been so precarious that to know that they would have something to eat for dinner and to know they would have a warm, dry place to sleep was a rarity in their lives. It put my complaints about the horrible food and lousy beds into perspective. It was one thing to know on an intellectual level that such people exist in our society—and I had seen glimpses of this side of the world—but to see this side of life up close on a daily basis was incredibly impactful.

— — —

On my very first visiting day (finally), my brother Larry came along with his wife and my yoga buddy, Colleen.

There is a long list of don'ts for visitors, but for anyone who doesn't understand the nature of the system, they might not seem serious. If a fan shows up at a stadium and the ushers tell him that he can't take his bottle of water inside, it gets thrown out. It is not that big a deal and no one demeans or threatens the fan for not knowing the water was forbidden.

Colleen set off the metal detector. She was wearing an underwire bra. She said the staff reacted as though she was trying to break me out of the prison. She was treated almost as a criminal herself for not knowing that she couldn't wear that bra inside. I would think a woman without a bra would create a bigger problem in a men's prison than a woman wearing the wrong bra. After, as Colleen described it, a humiliating dressing down by the guards, she remembered she had her yoga clothes in her car and had her sports bra in there. She ran out and did a quick change and was allowed to return.

I felt bad for my guests that they had to endure these humiliations. Every visit they had to pass through the metal detector and were subject to a pat down. Sometimes I think the guards did the pat downs just to further embarrass everyone.

Larry had been updating me on the phone and via emails, but he didn't want to tell me just how bad things were with Bob until he could do so in person. Although I had been preparing for the worst, it still hit me hard that I would likely never speak to Bob again. Recently, Bob and I had been getting close, and now our budding friendship would end while I was behind bars.

We were allowed very brief hugs under the very watchful eyes of the guards, but those fleeting touches meant a lot. I still had no idea when I'd be transferred or where, so I might have to make the warm memory of these encounters last for weeks or months.

One of the perks of visits was that there were vending machines in the visiting area. I was not allowed to touch the machines or money, but my visitors were allowed to use them. I was not a fan of junk food and never in the real world would have stooped so low as to have a disgusting microwaveable Philly cheese steak from a machine, but after the horrible food I had been eating upstairs, I don't think I ever had a sirloin steak or lobster tail in my life that tasted as good as that rubbery stale cuisine.

After visits, inmates were subject to a search, for fear our guests had tried to smuggle things in to us. These searches were a full strip, body-cavity type, but it was worth it to see my family and friends. I also couldn't help notice that although I was subject to the searches, the Latino or African American guys were definitely checked more closely, and they were usually made to cough a few extra times while they were bent over spreading their cheeks. There was definitely white privilege in the prison system; I doubt it was an institutional policy, but rather the choices of individual guards who were allowed a lot of leeway as far as how they treated prisoners.

Once the visit was over, I went to see my counselor to see if it might be possible to get a furlough to visit Bob or perhaps to attend his funeral, which now seemed imminent. Getting to see the counselor, like everything else, involved standing in line. The counselor only came twice a week for ninety minutes, which meant everyone who had any issues had to try to fit it into his narrow window. The frustration would rise in the line if someone was taking too long and time was about to run out. If the counselor was understanding, he might actually let an inmate use his phone, but if he did that it meant others had to wait even longer to see him.

My counselor, although not unsympathetic, was not exactly moved by my plight either. He told me I would likely be transferred soon, and that it was highly unlikely that I would be given leave before that happened. He also hinted that I was destined for a prison camp rather than an actual prison. He implied he wasn't supposed to say anything at all about my possible destination, but perhaps he felt sorry for me, given the situation with my brother.

In the meantime, as Christmas drew nearer, I wanted to stay in touch via the less-than-great email system. It meant a lot to me that my messages were getting shared among my friends. I had already met a few guys, and would meet many more, who had no one on the outside to care about them enough to write or visit. As much as it pained me to know that I was causing worry to my family, it also felt good to know they would care if something happened to me in here.

Dear Friends:

I hope this note finds you well and that you are taking some time to enjoy the holiday season. While there are no outward signs of Christmas here, we all know that Christmas isn't really about gifts or trimmings. The lack of commercial distractions here actually deepens the true meaning of the season. I take great comfort in this.

Crazy happenings here... a group of inmates was being transferred up from DC during dinner when one of the new inmates got into a fight because he didn't want the top bunk. He had to be subdued by the guards just like you see on those prison reality shows. It was insane. Then another inmate started yelling at the guard, who proceeded to lock us down from 5:30 PM till 6:00 AM the next morning.

As you probably have heard, I've been designated to a prison camp. Don't know when this will happen but think there's a chance it could happen before Xmas. It will be a welcome change moving to a minimum-security prison, where there will be more "space" and where I will definitely be working some type of job. Pay is $5.00 per month! Will let you know the details as soon as possible. I am ready to move. During the transfer I will not have access to phone or email for approx. 3 days so don't panic if I go silent. Think that when this portion of my sentence is over I will look back with great satisfaction as a period of deep growth. However, living here day to day has been one of the most challenging experiences in my life, yet one that I wouldn't trade.

Colleen sent me a picture book with hundreds of yoga poses. William, the young man mentioned in my previous update, borrowed the book and has taken it to bed with him the past 6 nights, and each morning comes to me asking to learn new poses (many poses I don't know myself). I've never seen a person so attracted and committed to learning yoga. We have started going deeper into breathing techniques and meditation.

Spending lots of time bouncing between a variety of books from history, mystery, to philosophy. I've been reading and thinking about the way different religions and philosophies deal with the concept of grace. There are common themes which connect all of us. Seems to me that each person is born with a sweet spot – free of expectation and regret, free of ambition and embarrassment, free of fear and worry – in essence a spot where we are touched with grace. Psychologists call this spot Psyche, theologians call it the Soul, Buddhists call it Dharma, Hindu masters call it Atman, and Jesus calls it Love. We all have this spot within us but it gets covered and suppressed as we deal with all life's tensions. If we drop the surface markers of identification, like where we work, how much $ we have, what we wear, etc., we can come back to that sweet spot of grace. Once we re-discover the grace within us, we should use it, hold it, cherish it, but most importantly let it guide you through good and bad times. Sorry for the rambling, but it sure makes me feel better. :)

Love & gratitude,
Mike

I wasn't sure which would be worse: spending Christmas in the stark conditions of the FDC where I at least knew a few people, or being transferred to a gentler facility in the next few days and spending Christmas where I knew no one.

The only notice anyone got was being told to pack his things, and then they came for him in the middle of the night. One night after I had arrived on the fourth floor, the door opened at about 3 a.m. and the cops came in and took my cellie. As scary as this part of the process would be, I also wanted to get it over with. I hadn't been there long enough to have accumulated much, but when I was ordered to assemble my things, my few belongings were all put in a box and I had to sign to verify the contents. I hoped to be able to sleep knowing that it might be a while before I could rest again, but I was too nervous to nod off, expecting the door to open at any moment with orders to move out. Eventually I did sleep and was surprised when morning came and I was still in my cell. No summons had come for me. Frustratingly, now I had nothing but the clothes on my back. No books, no toothbrush, sneakers, shaving kit—nothing. Everything I owned (in this new world) had been taken away.

All I could do was think about my situation and try to meditate and send some positive thoughts to Bob as I wondered how he was. Once again it was a moment to examine my life. Here I was starting the Christmas season without so much as a spare pair of underpants; I would have to look within myself for whatever might constitute the spirit of the season. That night I went to bed not knowing if this was my night, or if I would wait another day and half a night. Struggling to find sleep with so much on my mind, I felt like I had just nodded off when the cell door slammed open. It was my time.

Chapter Eight
Diesel Therapy

There is a fine line between depression and joy.
The human spirit is strong, but it can be broken if not nurtured.

It was two or three in the morning when I was ordered from my cell and into the common area. Two other men from the wing were also brought out.

We were taken to a holding area, and I was told to strip out of my jumpsuit, searched—including the humiliating part of bending over to spread my butt cheeks. I was given a paper jumpsuit and paper socks to put on. They started bringing people from other wings, and soon it looked like a bus station at rush hour.

As I waited my turn to be shackled, I heard a few of the men complain that their restraints were too tight and the guard putting them on said, "Tough shit." A few of the men tried to cock their wrists to make them larger in hopes of getting themselves a little more slack when they relaxed. This only seemed to provoke the CO and he put the shackles on extra tight. When my turn came, all I could do was submit.

There was about a foot of chain between my ankles so I could only take baby steps. In paper shoes that didn't fit well, I was afraid I might trip and if I did, with my hands shackled to my waist, there would be no way to break my fall.

The handcuffs were so tight that within a few minutes my hands were throbbing. The shackles were much tighter than they had been for the trip from the holding area beneath the courthouse, and this was going to be a much longer trip. How long, I had no idea. Some of the more experienced guys at the FDC had warned me that no matter how close the destination, these trips could take anywhere from one very long day to a week. Or more.

By about 4:30 a.m., everyone was shackled, and we were shuffled to another holding area to be processed and our IDs checked. By about 6 a.m., we were herded into the depot beneath the prison, where five buses waited. From the outside, they looked like ordinary school buses, but white instead of yellow. No markings said "Bureau of Prisons" or anything to indicate that these vehicles weren't taking students on a field trip or senior citizens on a junket to a casino in Atlantic City. I wondered how many times I had passed one of these buses on the Pennsylvania Turnpike or Garden State Parkway and had no idea as to the sorry state of the passengers inside.

The underground garage was freezing. We had no coats and our paper shoes and paper jumpsuits were inadequate for the December cold. I hoped we might be loaded onto the buses quickly, but as so often the case with the BOP, it was another instance of hurry up and wait. The cold breeze had my whole body shivering, but I knew that complaining was unlikely to improve the situation.

Some guys found friends in line and went to stand with them. Sometimes the cops didn't care that they did. Other times the inmates got split up and moved back to their place in line. No one was talking, so it wasn't as though they were catching up with their friends, but I guess it felt good to be in the proximity of someone they knew; if I had known anyone I suppose I'd have done the same.

I tried to focus on something other than being cold, and as I looked around, I almost started laughing when it struck me that if not for the paper prison outfits, it really did look like a SEPTA (Southeastern Pennsylvania Transportation Authority) transit terminal.

We probably stood there in the basement of the prison in the cold for half an hour. During this wait as well as for the rest of the journey, time became a strange concept. I had no watch, there were no clocks, they would feed us on their schedule, not on any normal pattern. In such an unfamiliar situation, it was hard to find an internal clock. I had been in enough boring meetings to have a concept of when the session was dragging into a second hour, but as in a dentist chair when pain can make fifteen minutes seem three hours long, here, time had no meaning and I had no reference points.

Finally we were allowed to begin boarding. The bus was heated and definitely warmer than the garage, but still far from a comfortable temperature. It appeared to be a standard school bus with a few modifications. Where the front row would have been was a cage in which a heavily armed guard sat. The driver was also protected in a cage. In the back was another guard who had a variety of weapons.

In the back was a toilet of sorts—completely open so the guards and everyone else could watch us do our business. Shackled as tightly as I was, it would have been hard to shimmy my pants down far enough to go, and I was likely to wet myself and the surrounding prisoners in the attempt. I couldn't even imagine what sort of contortions would have been necessary to do more than pee.

Some guys tried to sit with someone they knew. Others grunted or jerked their heads in greeting to friends as they shuffled down the aisle. Once again, I seemed to be the only person who knew no one.

I looked around to see if I recognized anyone. I didn't. I guess I needed to get to know more people in the system. For some reason, I felt safer near the guard, and sitting in the front would mean passing far fewer of the unhappy-looking men on board. Some were more than unhappy. One tattooed Latino was already going crazy, kicking and yelling obscenities. I practiced controlled breathing to calm myself down, but violent distractions like this were making it difficult to "enjoy the moment."

One of the guards, rapidly growing weary of this delay, drew his gun and pointed it at the man's head. Would he really have shot him? I doubt it, but apparently the angry prisoner didn't want to put that to the test. He settled down.

Eventually there were forty or more of us on board, and the bus pulled out into the early-morning light of downtown Philadelphia. Where my Diesel Therapy would end, I saw no point in trying to guess.

Most white-collar guys and nonviolent offenders didn't get Diesel Therapy at all. They self-reported to whatever prison camp or minimum-security penitentiary was to be their home. Most of the guys who got DT were either down a long time or were violent offenders who got moved around a lot, sometimes to break up gangs, sometimes apparently just to mess with them.

I was not exactly sure how these trips, whether by airplane or bus, got nicknamed Diesel Therapy, but with gallows humor it was said that it was the BOP's idea of therapy. It was quite a lesson in self-restraint to be able to sit for hours and do nothing. Nothing. No reading. No watching movies. Minimal talking. I couldn't even scratch an itch or adjust my boxers. There was no one to guide me through this therapy, and how I came out of it was up to me.

Joy. Surrender. True self.

At least I had my mantra and my meditation practice to help me cope. Some men, while clearly trying hard not so show fear, were actually in worse emotional shape than I was.

The bus started to smell of the nasty odor of dozens of men who hadn't been given a chance for frequent showers. Some guys (who were apparently used to DT) quickly fell asleep. As tired as I was, I didn't think that would be possible given my general discomfort and overall nervousness.

The story was—and again I wasn't sure what to believe—that years ago the prison authorities would let prisoners know where they were going and take them more or less directly there. Supposedly there was some sort of prison break attempt—the bus was ambushed and several marshals were killed. Now no prisoners knew their destinations or when they were leaving or where they were going. No one went directly from Point A to Point B, so anyone trying to follow or find someone couldn't.

There was also a bit of a shell game, in that several buses pulled out at once and headed different directions, so that anyone waiting and watching might still be thrown off the scent. There was no segregation on these buses: we had lightweight offenders like me on board (probably the only non-felon in the bunch), along with guys who had committed multiple murders and were doing life without parole.

I was close enough to the driver to hear him periodically checking in on the radio to let someone know our position and updating our estimated time of arrival.

— — —

Doing any physical yoga was out of the question, but I took simple breaths to calm down. I just had to make up my mind that it was good to be getting it over with before Christmas. And the sooner I moved, the sooner I could start building a life—such as it would be—for the next eight months.

We must have driven in circles or taken some circuitous route because although the first stop was at Fort Dix, New Jersey—what should have been about an hour's drive east of Philadelphia—it seemed to take several hours.

We drove in the gates of the federal penitentiary next to the Army base of Fort Dix. Inside, there was a huge bus terminal—like a large Greyhound station, but with everyone dressed in paper jumpsuits in the different colors based on their originating prisons. Clearly this was a rerouting point, where prisoners were swapped from bus to bus, bound for other destinations, as I had switched airplanes for countless flights.

They read off numbers and the men who were called got off. We stayed there for a couple of hours, waiting. Since no one communicated with us, there was no way of knowing if perhaps I was supposed to get off here as well—perhaps to be put on another bus, perhaps to be taken to a cell to spend the rest of my sentence here. All I could do was wait. We were on a bus service operated by the BOP, for unwilling passengers to destinations unknown.

After a while—again it was hard to tell how much time—a few men replaced those who had departed and the bus pulled out. The next drive took an hour or two. I had spent enough time in northern New Jersey to know that we were on our way to New York.

Our next stop was indeed lower Manhattan. It was hard to see from the bus, but it appeared that we were approaching Wall Street. Then we made a turn and drove under an office tower near the financial district. As with the FDC in Philadelphia, if I had passed this building prior to this visit, I had never noticed that this nondescript place was actually the Metropolitan Correctional Center (MCC).

Some of the guys seemed to enjoy some aspects of being out and seeing part of the world, even if the price they paid for that driving tour was being shackled in discomfort. For some, I'm sure this was their first visit to New York City, and they seemed excited to see it, if only from the bus. I was never much for random Sunday drives, but

I can only imagine that for guys who had seen the same walls for a decade or more, this trip was somewhat of a welcome change.

At the MCC, more people got off, more got on, and we sat for a few more hours. By now it was probably about 6 p.m., and we were each given one bologna sandwich. It was the only food we'd had all day so as bad as it was, I ate it. We were also each given one small cup of the watered-down orange drink. As we'd had no other liquid all day, I greedily consumed the drink.

From Manhattan we drove to an industrial section of Brooklyn. Here was another deceptively benign exterior concealing another prison in plain sight. It was shortly past dark now. At this stop, everyone was ordered off the bus.

As I was to discover was the routine at each overnight stop, we'd be taken off, photographed and fingerprinted, and there was no word as to how long I was staying. It felt good to get the shackles off; my hands and feet were painful, numb and tingly. I wondered if full feeling would ever return.

We got walked down a long hall and taken into a special area for prisoners in transit. I was locked in a cell with an Ecuadoran drug dealer who was lonely and eager to talk to someone. He said he had been in this holding area for days, locked in his cell twenty-three hours a day with no radio, no books, nothing with which to entertain himself. He had one jumpsuit and was only let out for one meal a day and a shower every few days. I wondered how such Spartan conditions were allowed in America. This seemed wrong on so many levels.

Enrique told me he was doing eight years for his drug offense, and then he'd be deported back to Ecuador. Like William, the clothing designer I had met at the FDC, Enrique made his detour into a crime seem like an accident, but one that was almost inevitable given where he came from. Again, I couldn't justify his crimes, but I had to wonder how I would fare if I was raised where and how these men had been. I couldn't help wonder, but for the grace of god... that could have been me.

By the time Enrique was talked out and I got to bed, as tired as I was, I had a hard time getting to sleep. There was a man on the bunk below me who had just shared his very personal story, and although I knew it was very unlikely I would ever see him again, I knew he would haunt my memory for a long time to come. I still hurt and felt uncomfortable and had the anxiety of what came next.

I found myself reexamining lots of my beliefs about how the prison system worked; sentencing for drug offenses and so many other things that were once theoretical subjects of newspaper articles were now the problems of a real person who was asleep four feet away from me.

I may have dozed off for a bit when the cell door opened about three in the morning. Once again we were shackled and made to wait in a cold underground garage. The sun was up and rush hour was starting when we got on the road again.

I couldn't help but wonder who plans to drive into Manhattan at rush hour? And gets lost. At first I thought the weird turns the driver was making were part of the plan to throw off anyone following us, but it became more apparent he was lost, as we circled some of the same blocks two or three times. My suspicions were confirmed when he asked the guard for directions. For two hours, we were lost in Manhattan. The driver was so desperate to get out of this traffic, he started asking inmates for directions—and they were giving him good directions; they wanted out of this mess as badly as the driver did.

I'll admit I've gotten lost in New York City. I think anyone who has tried to drive there has. But it's not my job to go there on a regular basis with a busload of people it was my duty to deliver safely to their destination in a timely manner. Does the BOP not have GPS? Or maps? This entire process would have been an absurd comedy if it wasn't so sad.

I tried to remember the concept of nondualism: the driver was no different than me. He didn't want to be in this situation either. Hating him, thinking bad thoughts about him, didn't change him. It only changed me. And not for the better. I started breathing again and calmed down.

— — —

In my early days of yoga, I was competitive. Not with anyone else, but with myself. If I could go this deeply into a pose yesterday, I had to go deeper today. I kept working until I could do a headstand. At some point, by proving to myself that I could do some of the more physically challenging poses, I had also liberated myself from needing to. Fine, I can do that, but now what?

Yoga, the kind of yoga I now wanted to do, happens internally. The movements are a means to an end, not an end in and of themselves. Now I had to practice yoga distilled down to nothing but the deepest spiritual part. No movement, just keen awareness of the present moment. An intimate practice on a prison bus bound for wherever. I found an odd liberation in being so confined, yet so spiritually free. How often in our busy lives are we made to sit still? Really still. In silence. No stimulation and no way to get up and seek any? How often do we take the time to go inward?

Driving back under the Manhattan prison woke me from my stillness. More numbers were called and men rose to debark. Other men were brought out to take their places and the bus was on the road again, this time heading out of New York and back into New Jersey.

We crossed New Jersey and into Pennsylvania. I'd watch as people pulled into a supermarket parking lot and I wondered if they could possibly appreciate the freedom they had to walk into that store and buy whatever they wanted for dinner. I wondered how I would feel the first time I had the chance to do that again. I was sure these people had no idea that this prison bus was driving through their community, taking men to stretches behind bars ranging from months to lifetimes. We stopped at a prison in Canaan to let off and take on more prisoners.

The many long business flights I took across the Pacific were annoying and tedious, but at least made tolerable by knowing where I was going and approximately when I'd arrive. Aside from the lack of any of the creature comforts an airline provides (I swore I'd never complain about bad airline food or a seat that didn't recline again), here the profound indifference to suffering on the part of the men who guarded us was in a way its own punishment. For the guards to do their jobs, it would be hard to practice any sort of nondualism. To do what they did, they had to very much try to keep up the barrier between *us* and *them*. I tried to remember the saying that I read in a book of Buddhist teachings: the opposite of what you believe is also true. No matter what we are sure of, there can always be another perspective, another way of looking at the same situation if we take the time to find and examine it.

I had been warned about Diesel Therapy, but as much as I thought I was prepared, it was much worse than I thought it would be. It was hard to keep from slipping into despair. But what did that mean anyway? That I would start to panic? That would change nothing. That I'd go crazy? That wasn't really going to happen. What would happen? All I could do was breathe and try to relax.

During the brief stop in Canaan, I had a sudden, urgent thought of Bob. I wondered if he was still alive or how I would know if he wasn't. I wanted to send as many positive thoughts as I could to him and hope—whether he was still in this world or had already passed into the next—that he was at peace; peace was something I knew he'd been missing for a long time.

The bus pulled out again and I tried to find my own peace. To release the worry about Bob and find my own calm again, not knowing if I was steeling myself for a few more hours or days. I also worried about my parents. I can't imagine the pain of losing a child— no matter how old the child. I felt bad that I was another source of worry for them at this time. I tortured my brain sometimes with how I might have spared them some of my trouble.

The next stop was not that far down the road and I was grateful. I truly wasn't sure how much longer I could keep it together. Somewhere near Pottsville, we pulled into a federal prison called Schuylkill. How could there be so many prisons? And we were only stopping at federal ones. I knew of a few prisons, but had no idea that the rural landscape of Pennsylvania and the urban skylines of Philadelphia and New York were replete with them.

Given that we were now less than two hours' drive from where I had started the previous morning, I had to wonder about the wasted time and gas and manpower in taking me to New Jersey and New York.

At Schuylkill, we were all ordered off the bus. Again the degrading intake procedures welcomed us to our new home. I woke the next morning still in the cell to which I had been assigned. It was past the hour at which I'd have been rousted had I been traveling that day. So I guessed I was to stay in Schuylkill, again with no way of knowing if this stop was for the night or for days or months.

But it would do no good to fret. One thing, I could at least stretch and do a little physical movement. I was let out for a brief evening meal and returned to my cell. More mindfulness. Some people paid large sums of money to do monastic retreats. I guess I should've been grateful I was getting mine for free.

The accountant in me still marveled at the amount of extra paperwork, let alone transportation costs, in needlessly moving people from Point A to Point B via Points L, E, and S. I knew from shipping manufacturing parts that every step—even necessary ones—added to the chances that something would get lost. I had heard stories of men getting lost in the system and had no doubt it happened.

The next day I also woke later than what would have been departure time if I was going anywhere. I guessed I was stuck here for another day. Or longer. Once again, I tried to surrender to the situation and made the best of it by practicing a bit of yoga. My body needed it after the confinement of the shackles. After so long on the buses, the added space of a tiny cell and the freedom to stretch and do a push-up seemed like a luxury.

Now I was to experience the frustration Enrique told me about in Brooklyn: twenty-three hours in a cell with nothing to do. Literally nothing. It felt good to be free of the bus and the shackles, but what did this freedom mean? Would I be spending the rest of my sentence here?

If I was staying, shouldn't I be processed in, given a uniform and a few other things? Maybe not.

In the middle of that night, I was awakened and told I was leaving. I wasn't sure if I should be relieved or worried.

We stopped at another prison along the way and dropped off some more people, and then drove another hour or so to Lewisburg Federal Penitentiary, arriving about 11 a.m. The gates of the infamous prison swung open and the bus rolled in.

Lewisburg first opened in 1932, and in an era when intimidation was more important than rehabilitation, it was built to look frightening. The builders succeeded: it did. The well-weathered red-brick buildings were surrounded by a high wall that was topped by barbed wire. A tower that seemed disproportionately tall loomed over the compound with an implied threat of snipers.

The prison was so high-tech for its time, it was written up in the magazine *Popular Science*. In 2013, Lewisburg got an "honorable mention" on *Mother Jones* magazine's list of America's Worst Prisons.

Over the years, the penitentiary had been home to many notable criminals and was the subject of the 1991 documentary, *Doing Time: Life Inside the Big House*, which was nominated for an Academy Award. During World War II, Lewisburg held civil rights activist and West Chester native, Bayard Rustin.

For whatever reason, central Pennsylvania has more prisons per square mile than any other region of the United States. That is saying a lot, given that the U.S. has the highest incarceration rate of any country on earth.

As unbelievable as it seemed to me, I was now one of America's 2.3 million incarcerated individuals. Among the many prisons in those beautiful rolling hills, two stand out: the State Correctional

Institute at Rockview, which was home to Pennsylvania's death house, and Lewisburg.

I sat on the bus and looked around at these frightening surroundings and wondered if I had what it would take to survive in a place that radiated as much pain as Lewisburg.

Once again I tensed, hoping my number would not be called to get off the bus inside the fierce-looking fences of this old federal pen. After little sleep and so much stress, my mind was playing tricks on me, and I was starting to fear this would be the final stop for me. Schuylkill was bad enough, but at least it was modern and less frightening. I didn't even want to spend a night here as we'd had in Brooklyn or Canaan, and I hadn't even seen the inside of the building yet.

I held my breath as they started calling numbers.

Chapter Nine
Cat and Mouse

Where I had felt despair, I feel hope.
Where I had felt lonely, I feel surrounded by loving support.
Where I had felt sorry for myself, I feel empowered.

Those unlucky men whose numbers came up disembarked to begin their sentences in the Big House. Among those called was a man who had been throwing a fit since we left Canaan, two hours earlier. Those two hours, although one of the shortest legs of the trip, had seemed the longest due to the commotion he was causing two seats in front of me.

When his number was called, he didn't get up. More guards were summoned and they had to drag him off the bus, with him fighting them the whole way. Once he was off the bus, we could hear the struggle continuing outside. I couldn't see what was going on, but the guy nearest the action was giving those of us on the bus updates as to the beating the man was taking. If anyone had filmed it, I am sure it would have been seen as police brutality, but the man had been resisting and fighting the cops the entire way and didn't seem any closer to complying.

It was one of the most intense things I had ever witnessed in my life, before or since my prison ordeal, and it was adding to my apprehension about getting off at this stop. I couldn't help wondering what ever happened to that man. I had left Philly with a man only being quieted at gunpoint, and now was welcomed to Lewisburg with another frightening scene.

I was very relieved when the bus started up again. The next leg of the trip was very short. The bus made a left out of the gate and drove down a slight hill to a small parking lot in front of what could have been a high school. In addition to the administration building, there were two, two-story brick buildings—the "units" in which five hundred men lived, and a one-story mustard-colored building that I would later find out was RDAP. It was off-limits to me and most other inmates, but housed the Resident Drug Addiction Program's participants.

Perhaps I was being picky or perhaps it was representative of the lack of care with which most things seemed to be done around the camp, but there was a sign near the road leading to RDAP that read "No Unauthorized Inmate's Beyond This Point." The unnecessary apostrophe was repeated on another identical sign. This institutional indifference to detail would be repeated in everything from trivial grammar mistakes to much larger frustrations with paperwork and other issues.

— — —

Finally, my number was called. What should have been a little more than a pleasant three-hour drive from Philadelphia to Lewisburg had taken four grueling days. It was about noon when I stepped off the bus and squinted in the sunlight at what had been presumed by many to be my likely final destination.

The Lewisburg Camp had been one of the prisons that was euphemistically called Club Fed. There was a time when certain white-collar criminals and lawbreaking government officials were sent to prison camps that were cleaner, nicer, and had many more amenities including better food, volleyball, and horseback riding. I was to learn that Lewisburg once boasted a salad bar and each inmate had his own cubicle. I am not sure how much truth there was in those stories, but now it was certainly not a vacation resort.

I got off the bus and took a breath. A chair had been brought out to the parking lot and I was told to sit down. As one CO watched over me, another cop removed the shackles from my ankles, and then my wrists, and finally removed the chain from around my waist. It was cold, but it felt so good to be unfettered that I didn't even notice the near-freezing temperature. It was such a great feeling, emotionally and physically, to be unchained in the sunshine. Like the old saying about hitting yourself in the head with a hammer: it feels so good when you stop.

I looked around and realized there were no fences. None. I could have made a run for it across the parking lot. I don't think I would have made it far, but it did seem odd to be so free after over a month behind barbed wire. I went into the building as directed, and a cop told me to go into the next room and wait to be called. He was one of the few nice guards I was to encounter through this entire process. He at least was trying to be somewhat friendly, which was a nice change after the cold, harsh treatment we'd been receiving.

In the next room there was no one. It seemed weird to be left unsupervised after so long under close guard. My fear level was falling rapidly. Until it started going down, I didn't realize that in spite of all of the mind/body work I'd been doing, I still had been at some level of alert and anxiety since I had been taken into custody five weeks earlier. My breathing was getting easier and my muscles loosened. It was obvious that this was a much lower-security prison, and that things would be taken at least a bit lighter here.

After all of the fresh arrivals from the bus were assembled in the room, one by one we were called into another room to be fingerprinted and photographed. The slow inefficiency of the process was now routine to me.

We then were called one at a time to go down the hall, where we were issued our uniforms. In contrast to the nicer cop in the outer room, the CO in charge of this process was clearly not happy with his job. It tested my chosen path of enlightenment not to call him an asshole; at times like this I would catch myself. Calling anyone—no matter how deserving—an asshole, was not a very yoga-like thought. I'd try to remind myself that every part of this experience—good, and especially bad—was a chance to just *be*, to be judgment free.

When I had time to reflect, I had to question why I judged the COs more harshly than I did my fellow prisoners. Were not these men and women trying to do a tough job? I knew that many of the inmates made poor life choices, or for a few life had made choices for them, which resulted in their current circumstances. Who was I to judge these guards or the choices that led them to this place?

I tried to be understanding, but it was difficult. This CO cared nothing about what sizes of anything I needed and issued me clothes and shoes that were all much too large. I think the boxers were XXXL. I could have turned around in them without them moving or fit my waist in one leg-hole of them. I tried to explain that and return the clothes to the two prisoners who were assisting with the issuance of uniform, but the prisoners didn't want to get this already-angry guard more upset, so they didn't exchange my things.

They did say that once I was settled I'd be able to exchange them. Not that the uniforms were really anything special. The khakis we were required to wear weren't actually bad. We looked like everyone worked for a utility company or delivered packages for a lesser-known parcel service. But their dullness was preferable to the much more prison-like jumpsuit to which I had become accustomed.

Not very helpfully and not very kindly, I was told my building and cubicle number—building 1, bunk 2—the place that would be my home for the foreseeable future. Unfortunately, no one told me where that was. I went out of the building in hopes of spotting a building number. It was my first good look at the camp.

There was a basketball court and a track. Way down the hill, on the road on which we had entered, was the housing area in which the majority of the prison's staff lived. Many of these houses would have fit right in on a World War II army base, although there were several modern ones as well, all two-story and well kept. In some ways, the situation of those employees was not that different from that of the people they guarded. They were isolated from town, living among the same people with whom they mingled day after day in the prison, with no fences, and the haunting presence of the Big House hovering above them. But those residents had one major distinction that set them apart from us: they were free to leave when they chose.

As I took in my surroundings, I saw three kittens frolicking in the grass. They were tumbling over each other and doing the typically delightful things that kittens do. I thought of the cats I'd owned over the years both as a child and as an adult. After the emotionally draining days of travel and my constant worry about my brother and my own future, seeing these small animals was more than my overtaxed system could handle, and before I knew it, tears were rolling down my cheeks. I'm not the kind of guy who cries easily. I don't cry at sad movies or even tragic life events. But these were a different sort of tears. Tears of release, resignation, acceptance, mingled with sadness and even joy for those kittens.

Joy. Surrender. True self.

Crying would hardly be a good first impression in a prison, but I couldn't stop myself. I realized that these creatures had found a way to not only survive, but to be happy in a prison. In their minds they must have thought they were free. All of the pent-up longing for a view of grass and sky from weeks in the FDC made this little taste of freedom overwhelming. I resolved that if they could somehow make it in here, I could as well. Soft start or not, I would find a way to survive and maybe even thrive in this horrible place.

Part of the practice of yoga is to be present: embrace the moment; don't worry about the past or the future. Just be where I am right now, doing what I am doing. I was enjoying that moment with the cats. The last five weeks or four days of hell didn't matter. The eight months ahead didn't matter. I am here in this moment with these kittens. They are happy, and for this moment, I am happy. And even in this place, there were things to be happy about and thankful for. My hope was to get a camp; I got it. The camp I hoped I'd get. I saw grass. I saw people walking around unconfined by concertina razor wire. I was thinking how precious this moment was to me. I was ready for whatever came next. I had a fresh hope that I could face all that was ahead.

— — —

I was carrying my new uniforms and still in my paper jumpsuit, so everyone recognized me as a newbie. An inmate walked by, and I asked him if he knew the location of my assigned space. When I told him, he asked if I was sure that was my number. I'd later find out why he was surprised: I was going to be the third man assigned to a cubicle that had only held two.

He took me to a large room with about fifteen cubicles down each side. The ceiling was about nine feet high and the cubicle walls went up about five feet, so I could look across the entire cubicle farm and see the heads of everyone who was standing up.

I met my new bunkies. At Lewisburg, we didn't have cells as we had at the FDC, so the terms cellmate or cellie didn't seem quite accurate, and "cubicle mate" sounded as though we were coworkers, so bunkie was the preferred term for those with whom we shared our small living space.

The cubicle was small, having been designed to hold one person. Aside from the areas occupied by the bunks, the floor space was about five feet by seven feet. Prison overcrowding now had most of these cubicles holding three people. All of the inmates were supposed to be equal, but I was learning that some of the prisoners were more equal than others. It was hard to know for sure why some got special treatment, while others got more negative attention from the cops.

One who got special treatment of the positive sort was my bunkie, Bill Majors. Because of his military last name and imposing stature, Bill was commonly known as "Sarge." Sarge was down a long time; he had been in about four years and is still there as far as I know. He was in his late sixties and had been a big-time lawyer in New York City. For some reason, his lofty status from the outside had followed him into Lewisburg, and he pretty much got whatever he wanted, within reason—he was still an inmate. I wasn't quite sure why, but I wasn't in a position to question anything. One of Sarge's privileges was that he had to share his limited space with only one other bunkie. Then I arrived and was assigned to his cubicle. And it clearly was Sarge's cubicle, only shared by Steve.

Sarge was a vegetarian and he worked in the kitchen, where he got the pick of the vegetables when they arrived. He used to eat whole, raw peppers the way most people would eat apples—just taking big bites out of them. We didn't get a lot of high-quality produce in prison, so coming by anything fresh and juicy was a real treat. I soon learned to crave canned peas as about the only vegetable with consistent, if marginal, quality.

At one time, the Lewisburg Camp had a large farm of its own, worked by the inmates. The place was surrounded by hundreds of acres of prime Pennsylvania farmland, so it made sense. Apparently the prisoners stole most of the harvest for their own personal consumption, leaving little to be sold as it was intended to be. Now the prison camp's main industry was cell phone recycling, which created its own ludicrous problems.

Bill Majors was a big man, probably six-foot-six or more, with a ponytail. The rumor—and whether these stories came from the individual himself or from others, I had learned to take them with a good deal of skepticism—was that Bill had been laundering money for the Mafia, got caught, and rather than implicate anyone else, had taken the full fall.

Sarge, like most of the guys at Lewisburg, was known almost exclusively by his nickname. When I was on the high school baseball team, we all had nicknames (mine was Hugs) and when I lived with eight other guys my junior year at Villanova, five of us were named Mike, so we each had to adopt a nickname; I went back to being Hugs. At Lewisburg, I would get to know everyone by the nicknames and sometimes never learned their real names. Steve might have been the only man in the place who didn't have a nickname.

As the newbie, I was given the top bunk. Sarge clearly resented having a third person in his small allotment of personal space.

After a while I began to read the subtext; apparently Sarge had upset someone in the administration and as part of busting his chops, they gave him another bunkie. Had they wanted to punish him too badly, they would have assigned him a bunkie of a different race.

One of the hardest things I had to get used to was how racially oriented so many things in prison were. As the father of a biracial daughter, it was hard for me to see race as a defining characteristic of a person, but in prison that seemed to be a big determinant for everything. In the tighter spaces of the FDC and with so many more men of color, there was less segregation. There had to be.

At Lewisburg there were almost no mixed-raced cubicles. Almost every cubicle was all-white or all-African American or all-Latino. At meals, each race tended to gravitate together at tables. At least Sarge couldn't hold my race against me. I don't think he was a racist sort of person, but breaking the color barrier would just have been another slap in the face to a guy who already resented having to have someone else in his cubicle. I am sure the guards assigned people bad roommates on purpose to punish them. I wasn't assumed to be a bad roommate, just another body crowded into what was too little space for one large adult, let alone two additional people.

While Sarge was giving me the cold shoulder, Steve was friendly and offered to be my tour guide to the strange new land of the

Lewisburg Camp. It seemed to me that some prison official should have told the new arrivals how this world worked, but none of them seemed inclined to do that. The excuse for a lot of things those first few days was, "It's Christmas, we're short staffed," or "That office is closed for the holidays." I had arrived at the Philadelphia FDC right at Thanksgiving and had received that same excuse for their minimal level of functioning.

Steve did a good job of explaining the "rules" and protocols of the camp and the invisible lines I dared cross at my own peril. Above all, it was clear we were never to snitch and never do anything to jeopardize or imperil our bunkies. Steve said he'd try to keep an eye on me for a few days to make sure I didn't commit any transgressions, but that I had better catch on quickly because he wouldn't be able to watch out for me forever, and I'd have to learn to sink or swim on my own. He didn't say this unkindly; it was just the stark reality of where we were.

He explained the "shot" system. Cops could write a prisoner up for an offense. There were different levels of infractions, and earning a certain number of demerits could earn you anything from a minor loss of privileges to a trip to the Big House.

I already knew it was verboten to ask what anyone was in for, or for how long, but at some point I found out that Steve was doing two years. He ran an HR staffing business and had "forgotten" to pay his taxes.

Steve was very kind to me. He was in the prison's education department and suggested I try to get a job there as well, teaching pre-GED classes. A few days later, once Steve was sure I'd be a good fit, he also invited me to be part of his card-playing group, where I'd meet some other guys who would become friends, or at least with whom I'd become friendly.

———

Steve seemed like a nice enough guy and that first afternoon, I desperately needed to open up a bit to someone to share my worry about my brother Bob. I wanted to ask someone how I could access a phone or email to get in touch with my family. I had no sooner told Steve my problems when I heard my name called over the P.A.

system, paging me to the chaplain's office. Steve gave me a knowing, but troubled look and told me how to find the chaplain.

The chaplain asked me to take a seat and then said, "I'm sorry, but we received word that your brother passed away this morning." I could only nod. The chaplain let me use his phone to call my family.

I had heard that there could be furloughs from prison—especially from a minimum- security camp—for family emergencies. I asked how that could be arranged and the chaplain said I could apply, but since I had just arrived and it being the holidays, he doubted my request would be approved.

As I walked back to my cubicle, an amazing thing happened: men I didn't even know expressed condolences for my loss. I was taken aback. How did they know? Weren't these supposed to be criminals? But they were all very sympathetic.

One large man in particular approached me. Just his size was intimidating, and I could see him getting cast as an enforcer on *The Sopranos* or *Boardwalk Empire*. He had a New Jersey accent, but his voice was gentle as he said, "I'm so sorry to hear about your brother." I asked him how he knew and he said, "Steve told a few of us how sick your brother was, and a page to the chaplain's office is only ever bad news. Especially by name instead of number. We just assumed."

He introduced himself by name and added, "But everyone around here calls me Bull." He told me his mother had died since he had been in Lewisburg, so he could understand how hard it was to lose someone close and feel so isolated from family at such a horrible time. He said he'd be happy to talk if I ever needed to. I would get to know Bull better in weeks to come.

When I returned to my cubicle, Steve also expressed his condolences and gave me a kind ear.

I was also greeted by the semi-official welcoming committee. It consisted of a few African American guys, all born-again Christians, who gave me shower shoes, toothpaste, shaving cream, shampoo—the essentials to tide me over until my money was transferred and I could buy my own items from the commissary. They made me aware of when Bible study and other religious services were held, but weren't pushy about it or trying to force religion on me. Nonetheless, Sarge resented them, as he resented anything to do with religion in any form. I would soon watch him engage in lively debate with some of the resident religious fanatics.

Later I found out that Bob had died at 6:45 that morning. It would have been about the time I was getting on the bus, when I suddenly had a very strong thought of him.

The chaplain had said that I could apply to the manager for a furlough. The manager was neither terribly sympathetic nor cruel; again I encountered the bored indifference that seemed common among the staff. "You just got here. Without a track record, we have no reason to trust you. You'll have to earn trust. And you don't have a very long sentence and will be out before long anyway." He was not happy that I had filled out the forms, which I had already been warned would not be approved, and now he had to formally respond. "You're here for a misdemeanor. No first offender gets prison time for a misdemeanor. The judge was trying to send a message by not letting you self-report." He made it seem like I was a dangerous criminal who would warrant close watching.

After learning I wouldn't be getting a furlough, I sent an email that I asked my sister to read at Bob's funeral.

> Where do I start to talk about Bob? First and foremost, my heart hurts for him, yet I know, I think we all know, that this was probably for the best. It was difficult watching him slowly decline these past 3 years. Bob was a hard person to get to know... He was outwardly quiet, a minimalist, and somewhat introverted. For those who really knew him, he was gentle, smart, caring and the most honest person I've ever known. I was fortunate to spend quality time with him and really feel our relationship evolved from a brother to a brother AND friend. We talked about business, politics, coin collecting, music, compared notes on our predicaments, and even talked about women. He

always said that he was too stuck in his ways and too shy for any woman to put up with him.

While he was in and out of hospitals, nursing homes, our house, dialysis, and physical therapy, he was always kind, pleasant, and complimentary to all the staff—to the doctors, nurses' aides, janitors—everyone. Even when he was in great pain, he was nice to everyone. It was part of his nature, part of his DNA. Yes, he was stubborn, yes he was non-social, but his heart and life were pure. He never wished harm on anyone and his word was as good as gold.

I am trying to appreciate the fact that he's in a better place and would like to honor him by remembering all his good attributes. Of course, we'd like him still to be here, happy and healthy, but we do not control life's events. The sadness is real and deep, but let's choose to remember him in the most positive way.

I believe Bob was put through enough in this life and was ready to leave. He left for a better place.

God bless Bob and all of us.

Chapter Ten
This Isn't Club Fed

It's easy to be grateful climbing up the mountain,
but what defines a man is how grateful he is as he tumbles back down.

Christmas in prison is not merry. No one was in a joyful frame of mind. Except me. Not that I was exactly happy, but I really was trying to find joy and there were things to be joyful about. Everything, even misery, is relative: I was not at the FDC, here the food was better, I had a lot more freedom, and the atmosphere was decidedly less tense. Although still far from a resort community, I was no longer terrified of almost everyone around me—guards and prisoners alike. Things like my yoga state of mind and the kittens helped me see the positive side of even this very negative place.

Paper Christmas trees and other decorations seemed more pathetic than cheerful, and too many men seemed to try to pin too much hope on them for their holiday spirit. The whole place had a depressing pall hanging over it.

In spite of the very recent loss of my brother, I was actually doing okay. His death had been expected for so long, and he clearly didn't want to live in his deteriorating state any longer, that I had already made peace with his passing. I tried to look within myself to find the deeper meaning of inner peace and goodwill toward men. I was never much into gifts, so not having presents didn't bother me at all. However, Christmas can be hard on anyone who is isolated from their families for the holidays for any reason, and being incarcerated intensified all of that. I witnessed many men plunge into despair.

I tried to share many of my feelings and experiences in a long email that I asked Jenny and Colleen to pass along to all who were interested.

The Lewisburg Camp is a welcomed change from the FDC. This should be my home for the next 8 months.

I no longer have to wear a jumpsuit as we all wear khakis and button shirts. Not quite Macy's styling but much more comfortable than before. The few personal items from Phila (radio, sneakers, shaving cream, books, etc.) are supposed to be sent here, but it will take 3 weeks (again our efficient gov. at work). I've learned how to trade for stuff here. I have traded future purchases of tuna fish for sneakers, T-shirt, and gym pants so I can at least work out. Commissary will not be available until Jan 4th so I am in effect trading "futures."

I'm trying to find a job that will be a good fit. I am hoping to teach GED students. It's not a high paying job ($5 per month!) but think it would be good to do.

The best part here is definitely not being locked in a cell. We are allowed to walk around the compound (4 buildings on about 15 acres) within limits. There is a decent gym plus a track and softball field... definitely not the YMCA but 1000% better than where I was. There are a lot of white-collar guys, drug rehab, and long-term criminals who are deemed to be nonviolent. Any rule violation earns a trip to the "hole," a lockdown cell at the maximum security prison 100 yards away. I was briefly there on Thursday and it's a godforsaken place...enough to scare anyone straight!! My roommates seem good... both a little older (which is a good thing).

During the lockup, I had a lot of time to think and would like to share some thoughts: In my previous updates I use the term "surrender"... let me expand:

In my mind, surrender should be a positive thing, not a sign of weakness, nor meaning to give up. For example, being confined for such a long time can cause depression, but if you accept your situation you can put it into perspective and look at the positives. In this situation I was able to (a) practice listening skills with cellmate, (b) practice meditation and breathing techniques, (c) learn about a side of life most of us would never experience or understand, (d) appreciate that as bad as it was I was relatively safe and got fed 3 times a day, (e) continued appreciation for the small things in life (like a shower and shave). Upon arriving at camp, just after the shackles were taken off, I saw 3 kittens and cried with joy.

With Bob, surrender means appreciating that he's in a better place and honoring him by remembering all his good attributes. Of course we'd like him to still be here, happy and healthy, but we do not control life's events. Having spent quality time with him causes me no guilt upon his passing. For sure the sadness is real and deep, but let's choose to remember him in a positive way.

I sincerely wish you a joyful day. Please take a moment to give thanks for all that you have. Think beyond the gifts and enjoy each bite of food, really listen to your family/spouse...in essence, enjoy each moment.

Love & gratitude,
Mike

My friends and family seemed to want to share this experience with me. When you are stripped of everything, your position, your income, your house, your family, even your own clothes, you have the chance to find out who you really are at your core.

So often in life—too often, perhaps—we view other people as their trappings. What do we ask people when we meet them—what do you do for a living? We judge them by the car they drive, the neighborhood in which they live, by their spouse and children—or lack thereof.

Here I was just Mike, with no wife or job or house to hide behind. It's a rare opportunity and I wanted to make the most of it.

I didn't know how many people were getting my emails, or as I started calling them, "my blogs," but from the responses I got there were quite a few, and the number soon expanded. Since the list of people from whom I could receive emails was limited, many responded via snail mail. It made me feel good to hear back from those outside, and I liked getting paper letters so I could reread them. Jenny or Colleen would also get emails from my informal support group and copy them into the prison system to send them to me.

It's easy to be grateful as you climb the mountain, but what really defines a person is how they react on their way down the mountain, when the fanfare isn't there. The cheering has stopped and now it's just the solo journey. How do you handle yourself when life goes against you?

Luckily I did have supportive friends, but I knew that for most of this trip I would be more alone than I ever had been in my life.

I'd heard of people who went the other way—from a camp to a FDC or higher-security prison—and I think that would be worse. To have gone from a relatively lax environment to a place where any wrong step could have serious, and possibly even fatal consequences, would have been a harder transition. There were still dangers here, to be sure, but I didn't feel like walking through the common area was threading my way through a minefield.

In prison, "white collar" and "white," as in Caucasian, were almost always synonymous, although in the camp I would meet one African American attorney from Philadelphia with whom, it turns out, I had friends in common. But other than him, most of the men who were Latino or black were not white-collar criminals. There were a few white guys in for nonwhite- collar crime, such as drugs. Overall, the camp was about 25 percent white.

It seemed that more of the Latinos and African Americans were down a long time. A common complaint is that there was a large disparity in sentencing for similar crimes based on race. A white guy was likely to get a year for possession of a small amount of drugs; a black guy could get ten years for possessing the same amount. I never did research on this, but from what I observed, it certainly seemed to be the case. Most of the black and Latino guys were there for drug offenses. Murders, rapists, and other criminals were generally in state prisons—rarely were their crimes federal as opposed to state.

I wrote another email, saying good-bye to one of the most challenging years of my life. I had never been one to keep a diary or journal, but while going through this time of major change, I found that sharing my thoughts provided a positive release, which provided space for finding perspective.

Dear Friends,

Greetings! Hard to believe that the year is coming to a close. Frankly, I am happy to move on to 2012!

I hope you had an enjoyable Christmas and are able to take some time off this week.

Last week was a difficult week dealing with the holiday, my brother's death, and missing his funeral on Tuesday. I know there will be many "low" days here, so am trying to take these feelings in stride.

Fortunately, mail finally started arriving from Phila. and I received many cards and letters Tuesday night, which really helped bring me back into a more balanced place. Again, thank you all for your thoughts, prayers, and well wishes. They really do make a difference.

I believe there is a fine line between falling into depression and remaining positive. You can clearly see it here, with some inmates making the best of their confinement by working, reading, writing, volunteering to run programs, and working out. They are engaged in lively discussion about politics, current events, etc. Other inmates have a blank look in their eyes and constantly complain about their situation, corruption of the legal system, loss of money, liberty, and family. While I happen to agree with most of their opinions, I don't think we can let ourselves get obsessed with it. Of course it's easier for me to say this. Many inmates have been here for more than 3 years (one of my bunk mates has been here for 7 years already, with 7 more to go!). Like I said, there is a fine line between normalcy and depression.

The days have been long and I'm looking forward to getting a job when the staff returns from the holidays. I met with the education dept. head and counselor and will most likely teach GED students. Hope to hear confirmation late next week. I would teach 3 small classes, each one 1 1/2 hours long, and will probably start with the pre-GED students, i.e. illiterate inmates.

Interesting to see the dichotomy of people here, with lots of well-educated white-collar people alongside many uneducated people across many races.

Kind of shocking to see illiteracy close up. How can these people ever hope to become productive without the basic tools of reading and writing (especially coming out of prison, where they already have 2 strikes against them)? I will also work with a small team to develop and run a job development program/workshop for inmates who are about to reenter society. Their workshops are held quarterly. Will keep you informed as things progress.

While I haven't seen or felt any physical threats, the mental anguish is all around. I assume that is part of the prison experience. Some workers resent the fact that we are not locked up and use mental intimidation as a means of control. I know we are here to be punished, but still am amazed at the total lack of compassion by anyone working here. Believe me, I'm grateful to be here but can assure you that this is still prison—not Club Fed. Saw the guards drag 3 inmates out of camp and into the big house into the "hole" for 60 days because they were caught using cell phones. I have no interest in violating any rules!!!

Love & gratitude,
Mike

One of the hardest things to come to terms with was my relationship to the guards. So many of them seemed angry all of the time: they seemed angry at us, their jobs, their supervisors, and at life in general. I later read in Forbes Magazine that "corrections officer" was number seven on their top-ten list of worst jobs in America. And I can believe it. Far more than the "criminals" with whom I was surrounded, it was a challenge to be empathetic toward the guards, and I struggled to maintain the belief that under our contrasting uniforms, we were all the same.

And I thought better of the COs than most of the prisoners. Most of the inmates harbored major resentment. The white-collar guys saw the guards as poor white guys who couldn't get on to a real police force and had to settle for this. The inmates joked that these guys would have been mall cops, except there were no malls around. The term most inmates used for the guards was "cop," and the "fake-" or "renta-" or "mall-" was implied in front of the word when they said it.

The thought was that they not only weren't good enough to make the police force, but they also weren't even good enough to be guards at the penitentiary up the hill. Most of our cops were out of shape, and guys joked about them needing to lord it over us because they were henpecked at home in the trailer park. The jokes were cruel and reminded me of junior high bullying, but the guards seemed to somehow invite it.

Whether motivated by profound indifference or petty power, the cops knew there wasn't going to be a customer satisfaction survey, so they had no incentive to get better. Rehabilitation didn't seem to be in their mission statement, so very few saw that as any part of their role.

I constantly found myself evaluating the performance of the guards and administrators as if I was still a COO looking for "continuous process improvements." Sadly, "process improvement" and the BOP don't fit in the same sentence. The way things were run would never have been acceptable in the real world—the incompetence in this alternate reality where there was no accountability. Here I was surrounded by convicted felons, but still I took most of my frustration out against "management," not the people who broke the law.

Some of the other guys and I eventually started a list of improvements we'd have made if we ran the zoo. The irony was that if these changes were implemented, it would have made life less fun for the inmates. Here's what we came up with:

a) In making their rounds, the cops always followed the same process and always came through the housing units at the same time every night: unit 1 at midnight, 2 a.m., and 4 a.m.; unit 2 at 12:30, 2:30, and 4:30. They should've mixed up the sequence and timing of their rounds to keep us off guard. Many crazy things would happen before midnight, but suddenly just before 12, the entire unit was "sound asleep" as the COs came through.

b) The "surprise" shakedowns were almost never a surprise. The COs always came walking down the main path from the administrative office to the housing units, such that one of the inmate scouts would give us notice that the COs were coming our way, and so people had time to move or destroy their contraband. The COs could easily have circled around the admin building and come through the back door of the housing units to significantly reduce the scouts' ability to warn the rest of us.

c) Of course, all of this could be improved if they installed cameras in the housing units. Surprisingly, there were no cameras in the housing units, though there were cameras everywhere else.

Some COs were better than others and did seem to care. I almost wanted to be nice to them, but they were not allowed to fraternize, and any attempt to forge even a small relationship with any of them was likely to backfire, so I kept my distance.

The nonwhite and nonwhite-collar guys had a bigger problem. The COs were all white. There may have been a few black guards at the Big House up the hill, but in camp, the guards were all Caucasian and some were pretty obviously racist. Others just had no idea how to treat anyone who was different.

Time and time again, I would see that I and the other white guys were treated better and afforded more respect than our African American and Latino counterparts. But there were also a couple of guards who seemed to think that all of the white-collar guys had chauffeurs and private jets waiting for us on the outside, and these cops enjoyed seeing the "rich" guys taken down a notch. At the FDC, about half of the guards were black and seemed to have a different—which is not to say necessarily good—relationship with the inmates. I quickly learned which cops leaned which way, whom to ask if I ever needed some little favor, and whom to avoid if I was thinking of breaking even a trivial rule. Some cops seemed very fair and I never saw them treat anyone differently.

Chapter Eleven
I'll Gladly Pay You Two Fish Tuesday…

Transformation frees us from guilt and
allows our authentic self to shine.
By embracing discomfort rather than suppressing it,
we can access our true nature.

As part of my blog, I tried to explain the fascinating economy and resourcefulness of the inmates.

Still anxiously waiting for access to the commissary. Fortunately I've plugged into the underground economy to get a haircut, a plastic razor, used sneakers, and used gym shorts (size 3XL). So far my debt total is 15 packages of tuna, 15 packs of mackerel, and a book of stamps. I will gladly pay this off, as this is not the place to default on your debts! Inmates are really resourceful. They borrowed an iron (we are supposed to iron our pants) and were cooking cookies and burritos! Have no idea how they even figured out how to get ingredients to make cookies.

Most of the economy in prison was based on fish. As in mackerel. Inmates were not allowed to have cash. All we had was money deposited in an account from which were deducted any expenses we had for phone calls, emails, and commissary items. We weren't allowed access to the vending machines, so when I could finally get visitors, I encouraged them to bring change which they—but not I—could use to buy snacks. Every transaction in the underground economy was on the barter system, and the most common currency was fish—little foil packets of mackerel (or sometimes tuna)—the type sometimes sold in vending machines. These packets were one dollar each, which made for a convenient exchange rate. Postage stamps were sometimes also used as the exchange medium—again, something with a known exchange rate, as well as intrinsic value of their own—I could eat the fish and use the stamps.

In the free market economy, prices fluctuated with supply and demand. Sometimes too many guys would steal eggs from the kitchen and the price would go down. Without refrigeration, there was no way to keep them long, so it meant they had to sell them cheap or throw them out.

I owed a good many fish by the time my money finally showed up, but I was grateful for the loans, and as soon as I had money on account, I quickly paid off my debts. I didn't want to be known as a deadbeat. But I guess they also knew where to find me; I certainly wasn't going anywhere for a while.

My cubicle mates paid a poor Central-American guy to clean our cubicle. Of course I was willing to kick in my fair share toward getting this work done. The cubicle always had to be clean for inspection, but we weren't thrilled with the idea of doing it ourselves. The deal was that for two fish a week, the Latino guy would take care of it. My bunkies and I had outside sources of money, but this guy had no money in commissary, and this allowed him to get some currency—fish—with which he could trade for other needed items. I had to marvel at the way the system worked. In fact, I'd encourage someone to do their doctoral dissertation in economics on how prisons could serve as a microcosm for the creation of capitalism.

Some months later, the Latino guy raised his price to three fish. We cleaned our own space for a few weeks, until he lowered his price and we went back to hiring him. Amazing how the negotiations that take place between unions and management at factories all over the world also occurred in our little cubicle.

We were three well-read men with lots of books. Bill Majors, in particular, had lots of legal books, and law books were an exception to the rule on how many hardbacks we supposedly could have at any time. My locker was full of books, leaving no room for clothes, so I learned the trick of folding my clothes flat and putting them under my mattress.

I was lucky in that my bunkies and I all felt some pride in having a clean cubicle. It may not have been much, but it was the only home we had at the moment. Other cubicles were inhabited by three slobs and besides looking bad, it earned them the wrath of the cops—something I didn't want to invite.

— — —

One other weird sidelight of Lewisburg was crossing paths with more celebrities than I had encountered since my days at the Molly Pitcher Inn. Quite different circumstances.

I got to know one of the guys who was portrayed in the movie *Goodfellas*. Not that we ever became close friends, but eventually he came to a few of my yoga classes. He was getting up in years and still trying to stay active.

Actor Michael Douglas's son Cameron was at the Lewisburg Camp until just prior to my arrival. The story was that Cameron, who was in for a drug offense, had gotten caught with drugs smuggled in to him by a visitor. Once again, I wasn't sure what to believe of what I heard.

Another brush with celebrity that I appreciated started with Brian, a member of the card-playing group into which Steve had welcomed me. Brian was one of the saddest guys I was to encounter in my time at Lewisburg. He had a huge chip on his shoulder about how badly he was treated by the system and the world. What he said he was in for, and what others who had checked him out said he was in for, were two different things. He clearly had issues, so much so that some of the guys called him "Rain Man" after the character in the Dustin Hoffman/Tom Cruise movie.

Rain Man was taking all sorts of drugs for depression and anxiety, having to queue up for the pill line every day.

Rain Man had been at McKean Federal Prison before coming to Lewisburg. (Again, another penitentiary in Pennsylvania I knew nothing about—how could there be so many prisons around?)

At McKean, Rain Man made the acquaintance of actor Wesley Snipes. Snipes was doing three years for what was characterized in the press as "blatant income tax evasion." Rain Man told me that Snipes was big into yoga and, in an attempt to help him, gave the guy one of his favorite yoga books.

During our shared time at Lewisburg, I tried so many times in so many ways to get Rain Man to focus on something other than his pain, including trying to get him to join the meditation or discussion groups I eventually started, but to no avail. From what Rain Man said, apparently Snipes had done the same. Rain Man said he had no intention of doing yoga, but when he was transferred, Snipes let him keep the book, which he gave to me. I found it quite useful and kept it.

It has been said that a lot can be learned about living by watching someone die—this was certainly true of the lessons I took from Bob's passing. I could learn a lot about how to do my time by watching Rain Man, as a lesson in "don'ts." There is a saying: "You've got to do the time or the time is going to do you." The time was doing him. It may not be possible for some people to ever find happiness under these conditions, but at least we could make peace with our surroundings and not fight every indignity and injustice. His bitterness made it hard for him to make friends—lots of guys didn't even want to be around him, and of course that made him more alone, which in turn made him more lonely and bitter. It was not a good cycle, and one that I constantly resisted.

In my next blog, in addition to sharing celebrity gossip, I asked my friends to share an important communication:

I'm sure you saw the urgent message about not contacting people here to help track down books, forms, etc. This provides a slice of what it's like living here and a reminder that this is prison and the people working here are not here to serve me or you, they're here to make sure we serve our punishment time and to protect the public from us. Another example: after visiting with Jenny Saturday night the correctional officer lined us up to yell at us because some of the visitors were arriving early and were not parking in the right place. He threatened to write us up, which can lead to a 45-day trip across the street to the "hole." So it's not the threat of physical harm that one worries about; rather it's the mental and emotional intimidation. I'm trying not to be paranoid, but sometimes cringe when I hear the voice over the PA system.

One of my friends had sent me some books and then asked me if I received them. I told her I had not. She called the warden's office, as a customer would contact Amazon to ask about a missing order. She meant well, but again it was a case of not understanding how seriously minor things were taken here. I was called to the manager's office and told in no uncertain terms that they were never to get a phone call like that again. Who the hell did I think I was? All I could do was sit there and take the tongue-lashing. He had all of the power. If I was not properly contrite, he could have cut off all future packages to me. He could take away other privileges, limited though they were, and I didn't think I could survive without visits and phone calls. The prison system had no way of punishing my friends who called or people who parked in the wrong place, so it was the prisoners who would have to suffer, up to and including a trip to the hole if it came to that.

I had heard of visitors being sent away for the day for minor infractions and other visitors being banned permanently, not just for major things like smuggling in drugs, but other minor things, like excessive touching or being too scantily dressed.

Visits were my lifeline, and a source of excitement, but also of frustration and concern. There was a weird protocol around visits. Like most of the guys, I lived for visits. We'd get almost giddy when a visit was coming. Besides seeing loved ones, it was the only time we were allowed to eat vending machine food.

In the real world, there are shades of gray. The prison experience brings things into sharp focus: everything is black and white. I watched guys go from a euphoric high to an epic crash and burn. I had to embrace any opportunity to connect with the people I love. The definition of cruel and unusual punishment is denying people a human connection.

At first it seemed silly to me, but then I started to get it. Inmates would get dressed up, fix their hair, put on homemade aftershave lotion, and fuss like they were headed to their first junior high date. I soon understood why: we each wanted to feel like a person. The whole prison experience was so dehumanizing; this was one chance to be around people who knew me as Mike, not Mike the prisoner, or inmate #60419066. I wanted those few hours to feel special.

The cops would keep us waiting in the hall outside the visitation room, sometimes for an hour. We could see our guests drive in to the parking lot and knew it didn't take that long to process them in. There seemed to be no reason for the delay, but it was instead just more of the power play by the cops. We were in no position to complain—we knew it and the cops knew it. We tried to wait patiently. If anyone even questioned what the holdup was or pointed out they had seen their family arrive, the cops made the same excuse about being understaffed.

This small test of self-control was actually one of the bigger challenges to my desire to remain calm no matter the situation. It made no difference to the COs if they kept us waiting, but every minute was less time I could spend with my family and friends, who had come a long way to see me.

The other downside of the visits was the search that followed them. We could be stripped and made to spread our cheeks and cough. Some guys found it so humiliating they would forgo visits rather than subject themselves to the process. It was worth it for me to see my loved ones. The concern on the part of the COs, of course, was that our visitors had smuggled something in to us. Perhaps because I was not in for a drug offense, or perhaps because I was white, I was only strip searched once in all of the visits I had at Lewisburg; most of the time, I just got a cursory pat down.

On one visit, months into my sentence, my daughter Maria, knowing how desperate I was for real food, smuggled in French fries. She had been to lunch at Applebee's and kept three French fries that she managed to get past security and into the visiting room. She then bought a bag of pretzels and snuck the fries into the bag and passed the bag to me. Those cold fries were amazing! Of course, I had to be careful eating them so as not to get caught. In retrospect, it was really stupid to do it. The risk of her getting banned from ever visiting again, or me getting a shot or worse, wasn't worth the fries, but my childish desire for the delicious food overcame my usual reluctance to break the rules.

I always tried to have something planned for the rest of the day after a visit so I wouldn't fall into melancholy. I had seen it happen to too many guys: they got so high, then they fell so hard. I tried to be mindful that there were lots of people who didn't get visitors; one of my bunkies only got a visitor every few months. I was careful not to gloat about having had a visit and wouldn't talk too much about it, except to friends who asked. Sometimes people would see me dressed up, and they'd ask, "What did you have to eat? Anything new in the vending machines?"

— — —

Visits were heaven, but getting a good night's sleep was always a challenge. Pillows seemed to be in short supply at Lewisburg, and getting one was highly unlikely even in the underground market. I took a T-shirt and stuffed it full of clothes, and for the rest of my sentence, this improvised pillow had to do.

I had a mattress, if it could be called that. It was more like a camping pad (foam with a heavy, green, plastic covering). I never saw them bring in new mattresses, so when someone left, people would grab the mattress from the vacated bunk, and often someone who was leaving would swap their better mattress with a friend.

One of the other things that interfered with sleep, besides the noise from next door, was being so close to the bathroom that the light shone into our cubicle—and not everyone was quiet on their nocturnal trips to use the facilities. We were also near the phones so had to overhear conversations—often unpleasant ones—at very close range. Equally hard to sleep through were the calls with guys telling their girlfriends or wives in great detail what they want to do to them sexually when they got home.

The snoring of dozens of guys made it sound like army barracks. The snoring was hard to take, but the other thing I couldn't get used to was the farting. I grew up in an environment, and my own home and of course workplace, were no-fart zones. Not that I never farted, but I masked that necessary bodily function in front of my parents, daughters, or coworkers. There was a guy in the next cubicle who farted loudly all the time. During the day, there was usually enough ambient noise to cover it, but at night it seemed to reverberate in the quiet.

Neither ear plugs nor eye shades were available at the commissary. At the factory where some of the men worked, they had industrial yellow spongy ear plugs, and eventually a friend who worked there got me a pair. Some of the guys made some eyes shades out of socks or some other cloth. No one ever got enough sleep, which contributed to everyone's irritability and made it difficult to maintain a positive attitude.

Chapter Twelve
Cool Hand Mike

It's easy to dismiss "them" as being different from "us."
The experience to live and breathe in a diverse environment
has erased the line between the two.

I never dreamed I'd go to prison, have dinner with felons, or come to think of some drug dealers as friends. I always figured I'd be more likely to meet men like Jack Welch and Warren Buffet than gang leaders or anyone portrayed in *Goodfellas*. I had proved my worth in the business world, and knew I could fit in on any golf course or in any boardroom in the country, but I wasn't sure I'd be able to earn the respect of men who were from such diverse backgrounds and were, in so many ways, so different from me. I wasn't a guy with street cred until I earned it in prison.

Nondualism teaches there is no difference between Warren Buffet and drug dealers. The only difference is in circumstances, opportunities, and decisions. Deep down, we all want the same things: to be loved, to be accepted, to be happy.

Not since my days in grad school had I been forced to share such close quarters with people whose habits were so different from mine, and it was difficult at times not to become upset or say anything. But I knew I would have to choose my battles carefully. In such tight lodgings, we often had cultural differences, but I realized much of the posturing and bellicose strutting was really based on each person's own fears. Fear may manifest itself in anger or violence. When I remembered my mantra, I could find no place for petty grudges or to dwell on small aggravations. *Joy. Surrender. True Self.*

I had always been good about hitting the gym, and even more so during the purgatory years, and as poor as the conditions were at Lewisburg, they at least offered some opportunity to stay in shape. I became friends with an inmate who learned yoga through a correspondence course, and taught the one yoga class at the camp. He was excited that I had actually had formal training as a yoga instructor and was eager to learn from me, not to mention how glad he was to have found a qualified person to take over the class when he was released.

I didn't know it yet, but some seeds of what I could do to grow into achieving things were already taking root. And I continued to read everything I could get my hands on that might help me focus on the changes I felt happening within myself.

I came across this line from the book Radical Acceptance, by Tara Brock, PhD: "The curious paradox is that when I accept myself just as I am, then I can change."

Through the practice of yoga both in and out of prison, we have seen tremendous growth through self-acceptance. This transformation is hard to describe, but it is real, as people confront their demons, embrace their suffering, and become comfortable in their own skin. This transformation frees us from guilt and original sin, and allows our true nature to shine. In a small way I can feel this transformation happening. During my yoga classes, I constantly remind participants that "yoga is a means for relaxing in uncomfortable situations" be it at work, family crisis, or prison. By embracing the discomfort rather than suppressing it, we can access our true nature. This is a simple, elegant concept, yet one which we must constantly be aware of as we deal with life's events. We use the term "practicing yoga" for a good reason, as these basic principles need constant development and reinforcement to be fully internalized.

I didn't necessarily mean "original sin" in the Christian way. Catholics are especially big on that concept, and even people who no longer consider themselves Catholic often have lingering pangs of guilt that have nothing to do with anything they have done in their lives. Others carry different forms of "original sin"—a sense of guilt or unworthiness because their father was an alcoholic, or they were raised by an unwed mother. People often blame themselves for things far beyond their control.

Much guilt and shame is unwarranted, and even if someone has done something wrong, after he has done his best to make amends, what is the point of his continuing to beat himself up for whatever it is he's done? He can't move backward. He can only move forward from the place where he is now. He can do his best to improve and work to not repeat his mistakes, but keeping himself up at night, reexamining things that can't be undone is useless. That energy is better spent learning what to do better next time.

I was skeptical of many of the professed zealots in the camp. I know there were some very sincere, devout men practicing their chosen religion to the best of their ability, and many who were using their time to seek some answers. But many who preached overly loudly and claimed a close relationship with God chucked that attitude the moment no one was around. Surely they would go back to their sinful ways the minute they were out of camp and had no one to impress.

There were guys who were into religion but completely devoid of spirituality. There were guys who were very spiritual but had no distinct religion. I could see the difference between the two and was willing to help those I could, and hoped I could learn from them. We could find fellow travelers, but ultimately we each did our time alone. I was alone with my thoughts at 3 a.m., but no doubt similar worries tormented everyone.

———

In some respects, Sarge was on more of a warpath than a spiritual path. I had to laugh when I heard why Sarge was in so long. The story was that he got into a snit with the judge who apparently was going to give him five years, and Sarge flipped out and said, "Fine, why don't you just give me ten years!" So the judge did.

Many of the white-collar guys looked down their noses at guys who weren't white collar, regardless of their color. Not everyone was that way, but certainly many of them felt superior. Sometimes I would see those guys put in their place—not with violence, because guys who were down a long time knew better than to go that route. It was actually fun to see some "uneducated" street guy whittle down the ego of a Harvard MBA.

The interactions between classes and cultures were often entertaining. One night a couple of Wall Street guys were playing cards against a couple of the inner-city drug dealers, and one of the white-collar criminals was bragging that he used to make over $500,000 a year.

One of these "uneducated" black guys started laughing. The Ivy League guy wanted to know what was so funny and the drug dealer replied, "Shit....I used to make that every quarter. And I didn't pay any taxes on any of it! Think about it—I didn't declare a dime! I paid cash for a nice house for my mom."

I wasn't at Lewisburg long before many of the nonwhite-collar guys started coming to me for help and advice. They could see I would treat them as equals and that I'd be willing to help. I saw them as guys who just didn't get the breaks I did, including the good fortune to have a dad who worked his butt off to give me a good springboard in life.

Through my good family upbringing, good education, through work and through yoga, I had learned that anger and depression are not good ways to live. So many of these guys never had the chance to see there was another way—they grew up in a world with too little education and too much violence, so it was not surprising that intimidation was their go-to problem-solving tool.

It grounded me to let go of the petty stuff that was going on all around me, and while I had so many men leaning on me, I was fortunate to have my family and friends to keep me grounded.

Dear Friends,

Greetings. Hard to believe another week has passed. My bunkie told me that the days pass slowly but the weeks fast. Well this is true! I've been here over 8 weeks now (over 3 weeks in Lewisburg). Hope your new year is off to a good start.

I am starting with the pre-GED students and will begin testing them to check their literacy level, then place them in the appropriate course level. In the past week, 20 new inmates arrived, of which at least 4 are illiterate, so now there will be no shortage of students. I'm really looking forward to finally getting started. On Friday, I assisted with an employment development workshop which my bunkie and another inmate run. The other inmate is transferring to another location so I will take his place and co-run the 10-week workshop. This workshop is geared to inmates who will be released within the next six months, so they are very motivated to participate.

I wanted the time to pass quickly but also didn't want to dwell on how much time was left, so I didn't count the days. I kept track by months. One of my bunkies had a calendar and would X out each day until we finally asked him to take that freaking thing down. It seemed to take too long for another X to appear. But each month, we'd talk about "another month down," and people tended to count the holidays: "Only two more Christmases here."

Some of you may be bored with the constant mention of yoga, however it continues to be a major positive factor influencing my time here. I've been practicing on my own for several weeks now and have gained attention from a bunch of inmates. The Power Flow style I practice is different from what they are used to.

Several people have approached me inquiring about the philosophy, benefits and poses. It's been a wonderful way to meet people, and because this style is physically challenging, it's provided some "street credibility" with the other inmates. They want to learn how to do a hand stand, inverted pushups, crow, and tripod poses. I've been practicing to center myself and to focus on the positive, not to necessarily meet people.

They all want to continue and were amazed how good they felt afterwards. One guy said, "Now I understand why everyone is talking about yoga."

Beyond the asanas (poses), they were really receptive to the breathing techniques and talked about taking breathing control off the mat. Am constantly amazed how this simple concept can cut across so many cultural, racial, language, and economic differences and get to the core of who we are.

People talk about going inward and losing track that they are practicing in a loud gym. Some people cry, some are full of joy, while others "just feel good."

For a few inmates who want to go deeper I've started an informal book club where I share some of the books you have been so kind to send me. We've already had one conversation about Radical Acceptance with 2 other inmates.

Beyond all of this, I continue to keep myself centered and not let the negativity that surrounds this place get to me. Just like you, there are good days and bad days here. Recognizing and accepting this can take the edge off the pain; at least that's what I keep telling myself.

In the next cubicle there are 3 Latinos who speak little English. One of them, Fernando, popped his head into my cubicle and wanted to talk about yoga—he is self-taught and has been looking at pictures from a yoga book to figure out the poses. Fernando is one of the pre-GED students (though not my student) and asked me to help him understand the words in the book. He asked if it was ok to call me "yoga boy." I laughed and said, "of course." It's these little interactions that are so rewarding.

Two nights ago, two correctional officers came to Fernando's cubicle for a shakedown, where they tore the place apart looking for contraband and throwing stuff all over the place. They didn't find anything of substance but riled up the entire unit such that they were up all night yelling and talking. Sleep continues to be a challenge.

It's been interesting comparing inmates at the Phila Detention Center to the Lewisburg Camp. In Phila you would tend to see people whose crimes would be printed in the local section of the newspaper (i.e. murders, drugs, home invasions, guns). While here, you might find the crimes in the first section of the Wall Street Journal. Last week's Wall Street Journal had an article about a major insider stock trading bust with

50 people convicted: several of them are here and are people with whom I periodically eat dinner.

Received a letter last week from Health & Human Services from the dept. of the Office of the Inspector General stating that they have started the process of "excluding" me from doing business with any business associated with Medicaid or Medicare. In effect, this ends my career in health care.

While I knew this was coming, the actual notice affected me harder than I expected. Seems like this "no criminal intent misdemeanor" has become the gift which keeps on giving. It's time to finally leave this behind and move forward. Will use this time to sort out the next steps in life. Any of you hiring? :)

The unusual dynamics of prison show up in the strangest places, even at mass. The priest here is Father Pat from Nigeria, who also happens to be a correctional officer across the street in the "Big House."

Every Sunday before mass, he lectures us on a different topic ranging from politics to prison life. The strange thing is he uses these lectures to berate the attendees, telling us how ungrateful we are and how we are wasting our lives. He does this in the most un-Christian way. He also reminds us that he is a correctional officer first and a priest second. Then he's surprised when no one goes to confession!! What's even stranger is that once he begins mass, he delivers some of the best homilies I've ever heard. He has a brilliant understanding of the scriptures and their relevance to everyday life. Part of me is turned off by him and the other part is intrigued by this dualism. Another part of me enjoys the show as you never know what you'll get next.

I have enjoyed delving into the spiritual aspects of religions. Perhaps the austere environment has helped me to look beyond the fallible man-made rules and ceremonies which tend to divide us and prevent us from focusing on the greater message. I believe if we can pull ourselves out of the minutiae (racially, socially, culturally), we can find so much commonality in the spirituality that is core to many religions. I have used this forum to espouse some basic Buddhist principles. However, the same message can be seen in Christianity.

While the words may be different, the message is exactly the same. The reason I raise this topic is that there are so many diverse people here and it's easy to dismiss them as being different from us. While I wouldn't wish prison on anyone, the experience to live and breathe in a diverse environment has been a mind-opening experience.

Love & gratitude,
Mike

Colleen had sent me the *Prison Yoga Book* by James Fox. In addition to being great for explaining and illustrating yoga poses, it did a good job explaining the limitations and applications of yoga to the prison environment.

Fox's program had been going on at San Quentin for about a decade at this point, and he had learned many lessons that I was quickly learning for myself. He intended the book to guide prisoners who had no yoga experience. He charged people outside of prison for the book so he could afford to give it away to those who were behind bars. I was making five dollars a month, so if I hadn't had another source of income, it would have taken me two months to save up for a $10 book, assuming I didn't want any mackerel or snacks or razors in those months.

I asked Colleen if she would be my conduit to James, and of course she said yes.

Dear Mr. Fox,

Greetings. My name is Michael Huggins and I am currently an inmate at the Lewisburg Federal Prison Camp in Lewisburg, PA and am serving a 9-month sentence. Since I don't have internet access, my friend and yoga teacher, Colleen, is forwarding this message on my behalf. Prior to coming to prison, I taught yoga at several studios using a variety of styles but primarily focused on Power/Baptiste Flow (I have been practicing for over 10 years). In addition, I taught meditation mainly focused on the Yoga Nidra guided meditation philosophy.

Colleen was kind enough to mail a copy of your interview you gave with Sarah Greenberg from MindBodyGreen about the Prison Yoga Project. I am experiencing first-hand the power of yoga on inmates and have been sharing my thoughts with several friends (please refer to the extracts at the end of this message). In just 3 weeks here my personal yoga practice has evolved into 3 classes (twice a week) with 12 inmates. These inmates seem to be embracing not only the physical practice but also the breathing and inward looking aspects of yoga. I am currently trying to find a quiet space to start a Yoga Nidra meditation class.

Prior to coming to this institution, which is a prison camp, I spent a month at the maximum-security detention center in Philadelphia. During my stay there, 2 formal yoga classes evolved from people observing my personal practice. Most of the correctional officers were supportive of the program and provided access to the rec room where we could practice yoga and meditation.

I read with great interest the work you are doing with inmates and the "Give Back Yoga Foundation." Last year I attended a workshop with Beryl Bender Birch and continued to correspond with her, so I'm quite familiar with the wonderful activities of this nonprofit. In addition, I attended a workshop and support another program called Street Yoga (founded by Mark Lilly from Portland, OR). Working with Colleen, we set up two nonprofit yoga programs for disadvantaged kids for the Police Athletic League.

Over the past three years my career has been evolving from the business world toward giving back to the community. I have made the decision to focus my efforts working with inmates and/or disadvantaged people. Several of my friends work with local prisons in the Philadelphia area developing reentry programs and I plan to reach out to them upon my release.

I will be released in late Aug 2012 and was wondering if you were looking to expand the Prison Yoga Project and were looking for assistance (as a volunteer).

I was happy and excited when James answered Colleen. It was the beginning of a relationship with James and his program that lasts and grows to this day.

I continued to update my little fan club of supporters. Each time I sent a message, it was gratifying to get responses both via email and snail mail. Sometimes I still felt the need to vent my frustrations.

There are many little things that become a challenge here, like getting the car registered. We (I mean Jenny) are trying to figure out how I can sign the registration when I'm not allowed to have any formal documents sent here (other than legal documents sent through my lawyer) and Jenny can't bring anything with her during visitation. Same is true with preparing our taxes. We'll sort this out but all of these things add to the punishment of prison.

Jenny told me that my bank account was closed (with no notice) since I'm deemed a person of "disreputable character." Apparently the bank scans prison databases for inmates and closes accounts. Frustrating as we pay bills out of this account, so Jenny had to scramble to set up a different bank for bill paying. As I've said many times...this misdemeanor is the gift which keeps on giving.

I went to see my counselor to see if there was any way I could have the registration sent to him for me to sign since it couldn't come to me directly. I wanted to get it taken care of before it expired. Pennsylvania police are sticklers for little things like that. The counselor said, "Just have your wife sign your name."

I couldn't believe what I was hearing. Was he, a government official, actually advising me to ask my wife to commit forgery? I wanted to scream, but I knew better than to get angry or I'd never get what I wanted. I knew it wouldn't compute with him that I was actually very honest and hated to break the rules, so I tried to convince him that my wife's writing was nothing like mine—I still wrote with big loops as though I was trying to impress the nun in penmanship class.

After some begging, I finally arranged to have the registration mailed to him. I had to sign and seal it in front of him. He was really pissed off at me that I made him do extra work. The camp administration seemed to have a pathological aversion to any kind of paperwork.

Maybe it was a premonition or paranoia that I might not get to self-report and get all of my affairs in order, but I did as much as I could to prepare. I had set up a money market account with a large, well-known banking institution to do automatic bill pay. Apparently this bank does reviews of its customers, saw my recent conviction, decided I was a bad character risk, and cancelled my account with no notice. The next time I called home, Jenny told me that all of our bills were bouncing. It was weeks before she got a refund check from the closed account and in the meantime, I had to tell her where to find money to pay the bills. Soon thereafter I read in the Wall Street Journal that this same bank had paid an $800 million fine for laundering money for Iran. And I wanted to scream—I'm the disreputable character who isn't worthy of an account with them? I was never a violent person, but moments like this had me wanting to punch something or someone. I understood why some guys did. It was hard not to get angry when it seemed like things from minor inconveniences to major hassles kept coming at us from all sides.

Years later, reading *The Divide*, by *Rolling Stone* writer Matt Tiabbi, further aggravated my sense of injustice. In the book, he better articulates the sense of outrage I was feeling in Lewisburg. Tiabbi questioned, as I did, why homeless people who own nothing get prosecuted for petty crimes, while Wall Street crooks who stole billions and destroyed lives never went to jail. It was weird to think that of people who were becoming my friends in Lewisburg, but I was glad that at least some of the white-collar criminals—bankers who had ripped people off with fraudulent mortgages, and corrupt government officials who had taken bribes—were eating the same shitty food I was. We often made reference to the "unjust justice system" in our discussions in camp. It was apparent there were two sets of justice—one for the rich and another for poor people of color.

I still wrote about the odd moments of life in camp:

I continue to be fascinated by the interpersonal socio-economic dynamics of this place, from the vibrant underground economy to the interaction of diverse people.

Yesterday there was a re-enactment of the famous scene from the Paul Newman prison chain gang movie Cool Hand Luke, where he eats a couple dozen hard boiled eggs as a bet. An inmate here did the same thing using eggs "accumulated" by kitchen workers and other inmates bet on how many eggs he could down. Anything to pass the time.

I had seen the movie a few times in my life, and never in my wildest dreams did I think I would be in a prison to witness such a scene for real. But now I could almost imagine some of the more intransigent cops saying, "What we've got here is failure to communicate..."

Chapter Thirteen
Special White Guys

If we look beyond man-made rules and ceremonies,
which tend to divide us,
I believe we can find commonality in the spirituality
that is core to the human being.

Life without Paul Newman went on, and I continued to chronicle the craziness that was Lewisburg. At times I felt that I was part of a strange reality show, with no hope of being voted off the island. Yet journaling seemed to become another way to maintain some type of emotional and spiritual balance.

I've met several more high-profile white-collar inmates, including a CEO of a large regional bank out west, a managing director of a large NY hedge fund, a well-known stock trader, the CEO of a mortgage company, as well as more insider trading guys. There is also the VP of Manufacturing for a vitamin supplement company who got 3 years for violation of good manufacturing practices. Seems like I'm not the only one the FDA is going after.

While there is the protocol of "don't ask, don't tell," people are fairly open to describing their crimes.

While people have committed crimes and need to be punished, it seems a waste to society not to use the talent here to develop programs to help the unfortunate or uneducated.

For example, we could easily develop a basic financial education program to provide "financial literacy" (i.e. explaining exactly how credit card interest works, managing a checkbook, buying a car—lease vs. buy, etc.). There is no interest in developing these types of programs as the focus is strictly punishment. Society loses as the men who could benefit from such programs hit the streets unprepared to deal with the economic reality and are likely to fall back into destructive behavior. For the white-collar guys, they leave disillusioned with the system and lose their drive to be productive.

It is so clear to me that the system is driven by the economics of job preservation for prison workers, rather than the desire to rehab people. Another example: Lewisburg gets money for every student enrolled in GED, but there is no incentive for students to pass. The longer they stay in the program, the more money the prison gets. If they were serious about rehabilitation, there would be an incentive to get inmates to pass in a timely manner. Inmates who aren't motivated are allowed to sleep through class and we aren't allowed to do anything about it. I'm now understanding what the term "institutionalized" means. It's a disgrace, but there's not anything we can do, as the public is generally not sympathetic to complaints from criminals.

There were people trying to make a difference. My boss in the education department was fantastic. We called him Farmer Joe, because for all appearances that's what he was. He was a large man and looked like he had just gotten in from plowing the back forty.

For too many of the staff, compassion, respect, or empathy was hard to come by—yet these are precisely the things prisoners will need if their lives are to be any different when they get out. I especially felt bad for those men who did not have a good safety net waiting to catch them when they got released. The prison provided used, donated clothes and $35 upon release for those who had nothing. They would be dropped at the nearest bus station and that would be it. I didn't know what bus fare was from Lewisburg to Philly or Pittsburgh, but I am pretty sure that alone would've eaten up the poor guy's stipend. I wondered, if someone had no one to pick him up, no place to stay, and no one to buy him food for a while—what would life be like? Stealing was likely to look like the only option. I would try not to torment myself worrying about such things and try not to whine too much as I continued my emailing.

As part of my mantra to extract every bit of education I could from this unfortunate experience, I was learning about people and cultures and things I not only had never been exposed to but also didn't even know existed to seek out such experiences. I didn't even know what I did not know.

One of the other remarkable things I noticed was that with this many guys together with almost no women and little close supervision, they tended to revert to a junior-high locker room mentality regardless of background, education, ethnicity, or socioeconomic status. Maybe it was the lack of female contact that made so many guys obsess over women, and particularly certain parts of their anatomy. I found myself looking at photos and laughing at jokes and comments that would have appalled me in my real life. Magazines such as *Playboy* were banned as pornography, but exercise and yoga magazines which featured women in tight clothing were permitted; my copies of such magazines were passed around quite a bit, and I didn't think that most of the guys were looking at them for the articles. But I actually did read them for the articles and comment on them to my friends:

The December issue of Yoga Journal has an excellent article titled, "Is Yoga a Religion?"

This is an excellent discussion with input from an esteemed panel of yoga masters. I'd like to add my two cents: I believe yoga is a deeply spiritual discipline which emphasizes knowledge and direct experience at an individual level. However, yoga is not a belief system. For this reason, I believe the spiritual nature of yoga can be layered onto any religion to deepen the religious experience.

Many people believe yoga is similar to Hinduism or Buddhism, when in fact yoga predates both. The Classic 8 Limbs of yoga is a means for self-examination, for quieting the mind, and for finding joy in an uncomfortable situation—and a means to deal with suffering. It is not a directive to follow a specific belief or religion but an effective way to deepen your spirituality within your chosen religion.

Personally I see no conflict between yoga and any of the Western religions, although I'm not an expert in this area. Just one person's opinion.

The question of what religion yoga belongs to comes up time and again. A court in California had to rule on this after a group of Christian parents brought a suit against their school district for allowing yoga to be taught in the public high school, when all other religions were prohibited. The court ruled that yoga was not part of any religion or religious practice, but in Georgia, a school banned yoga as being "un-Christian."

After I got out, a woman who attended one of my trainings said she addressed this issue by saying, "Rabbis do yoga, Muslims do yoga, Catholic nuns do yoga, Hindus do yoga, atheists do yoga—so if it's a religion, what religion is it?"

I think if done properly, yoga can help anyone come to a deeper appreciation of their religion, whatever that may be—or no religion, if that is his or her choice. But it can definitely lead to spiritual awakenings if one is open to them.

Dear Friends,

Hard to believe that January is coming to a close. It's been a difficult week here as I seem to be stuck in a funk. Think it may have started Tuesday night when a weight fell on my head during a workout, causing what I believe is a mild concussion. I have a big lump on my head and lingering headaches. Fortunately, I was able to buy Aspirin at the commissary, which has helped. I refuse to see the physician's assistant. I have heard horror stories about the quality of healthcare here. Besides there's not much more that can be done.

This funk may be due to other things like the lack of privacy, lack of compassion, and selective enforcement of the rules. My cubicle, which was built for 1 person, houses 3 of us, and we must stand in a straight line during the standup counts as we can't fit standing shoulder to shoulder. There are no quiet spaces on the compound. The library has 2 tables and 10 chairs, but is regularly filled with at least 15 people. I would give anything for a few hours of quiet solitude. Things will get better in the spring as we'll be able to sit outside in the open space.

The opportunity to live in this melting pot of culture has been frequently mentioned in these updates. This generally has been a great experience... although not this week.

I've also mentioned how bad the food is... well it's gotten worse, as inmates and guards have been stealing food. Saturday night we were supposed to have "chili mac," which is lousy to begin with, but some inmates stole the ground beef so we had only macaroni. I returned to my housing unit to see inmates selling stuffed beef burritos. Very frustrating, especially as we get limited protein in our meals as they fill us up with starch... rice, bread, potatoes, macaroni, and beans.

I'm told that the guards are just as bad as the inmates. Yet, if we have 6 hardcover books we get into trouble!

The guards had to know what was going on. Sometimes, I would see guys walking away from the kitchen carrying large quantities of food. If I saw it, the guards had to. The food was bad to begin with, but to have guys skim the best of the bad was painful to watch. I don't know what the guards were getting out of this—some kind of kickback? But what did the men have to give the guards? And it was crazy because so many of the guards seemed to take such pleasure in busting our chops about the smallest things. Maybe it was just honor among thieves—we would see guards backing their pickup trucks up to the kitchen and loading up on food meant for prisoners.

There was one CO in particular who was petty and brutal—at breakfast he'd throw people out of the chow hall when time was up, whether they were done eating or not. The lines were so long to get food that people who were toward the back were often only left with a few minutes to wolf down their food. None of the other cops cared. If anyone talked in line, or looked at him wrong, he'd throw the offending party out of breakfast. I saw guys confront him, and then soon after they'd be sent to the SHU on a supposedly unrelated matter, but it happened too often to be a coincidence. I did my best not to cross him. Not that I was ever slovenly, but if I saw he was on duty,

I'd look myself over to make sure my uniform was up to his standards. There was a policy if anything was left over, we could go back for seconds, but he would dump the leftovers rather than let these hungry guys have seconds. So many of them couldn't afford any extra food from commissary, and were therefore starving most of the time. It was just cruel, and I felt so bad for the guys as they watched food go in the trash. A total pacifist myself, even I wanted to hit him, so for guys with anger issues—and there were a lot of them here—he was definitely pushing their buttons.

Ironically, most of the food belonged in the garbage. It was so disgusting it really wasn't suitable for human consumption. In fact, even the cats wouldn't eat most of it. Guys would steal food from the chow hall and with good intentions try to feed it to the kittens, but the cats were smart enough to refuse it. Other guys would actually buy fish just to feed the cats—they had grown that fond of the little fur balls.

I couldn't handle the bad meat, and for the most part became a vegetarian. I'd look down the food line and see what was being served. If it was gross—and it usually was—I'd tell the men who were spooning the slop that I was a vegetarian, which meant I'd get double helpings of the vegetables, but no meat. I never thought I'd consider canned peas a good dinner.

This particular CO was cruel beyond what the job required: he knew it and we knew it. But we also all knew no one was ever going to do anything about it. There were also a couple of really bad supervisors—sergeants—who would arbitrarily turn the TVs off. It was supposedly somewhere in the rules that they couldn't do that, but they knew no one would do anything about that either. It just seemed arbitrary and petty to torment men who already had so little. I felt fortunate that I was not dependent on TV for entertainment. I had my books, interesting companions for conversation, and my teaching and tutoring. But so many of the men were barely literate, and the TV was almost all they had. How was showing these men such small-time tyranny supposed to prepare them for life outside? Shut off the TV in a bar in the fourth quarter of an Eagles game and see what sort of a reaction occurs.

Many of the guards weren't bad and were just trying to do a thankless job. They weren't on a great career path and knew it, but even among the good ones, I never saw any who were happy or took joy in their job. How could they? Their job description was to enforce picayune rules over the dregs of society.

I would get angry and then try to remember my mantra—*Joy. Surrender. True self.*— and try to find a place in my heart for that seemingly heartless cop. There had to be some reason for him to be that way. What did I know of him and his life experience? He may have had dreams for his life and saw each wasted day as one having to watch us getting in the way of those dreams.

It wasn't like all of the cops tried to be difficult; there were other guards who tried to be nice while still keeping discipline and maintaining the barrier they had to between themselves and the prisoners. They weren't here to be our friends or do us any favors, but they would yell "last call" for seconds before dumping the food. They'd let people stay and finish eating instead of chasing them out at the end of meal time. We weren't supposed to take food from the chow hall, but many would let us go with a little something—I'd often take my banana and milk for later.

———

There were other problems with the cops as well. I was sort of surprised to see that there were female guards in a men's prison. Two in particular flirted with inmates very inappropriately. One CO had a reputation for making the lives miserable of anyone who rejected her flirtations.

A couple of the other female cops were actually quite attractive and the subject of many inappropriate comments on the part of the inmates. There was craziness on all sides, but I never heard of any of the men actually doing anything with a guard. We all knew that several of the COs were dating each other—while married to other people. With so much drama in front of us, did anyone really need to watch Jerry Springer?

There was a common expression: I know when I'm getting out— the guards are in prison for their whole careers. I tried not to let my blogs become unrelenting bitch sessions, but sometimes they did, and

I guess it was better that I vented to friends than to my fellow inmates or the COs.

The lack of compassion continues to be the singular most appalling aspect of this place. There are too many examples to list... here is just one: Brian (Rain Man) is one of the guys I play cards with. He's from South Carolina and is 2 years into a 5-year sentence. He has two children (10 & 12) and is in the middle of a divorce. Due to school and the travel distance, he only gets to see his kids once a year in July. Federal law states that inmates should be incarcerated no more than 500 miles away from their home. Brian's family lives literally 499 miles from Lewisburg (as the crow flies—it's more than 500 miles by car or plane), yet the case manager refuses to help him transfer to a camp, which would only be 2 hours from his family. The case manager said he would reconsider again next October! Brian has been an ideal inmate, never in trouble and is trying to be a good father while being in jail. For the life of me I can't understand why the case manager would be so cruel. Beyond that there is this sense of indifference to the pain and suffering this causes him and the negative impact this has on his children. Brian has slipped into depression for which he takes medication. Sad, sad, and totally avoidable. He's not trying to get out of his sentence, only have the ability to connect with his children. Cruel and unfortunately not unusual punishment.

And there were other stresses acting on all of us.

Been a crazy 8 days over at the Big House as 5 people were murdered, 3 by stabbing and 2 stomped to death. Also a guard was beat up and hospitalized. We had several more lockdowns here, but not as long as last week.

Sometimes we could actually hear screaming coming from the Big House. It was terrifying and sent chills down my spine. As though I didn't already have incentive to avoid going up the hill to the hole, these experiences reinforced that goal. The guard tower and the wall of the pen loomed over us, and as hard as it was to avoid looking at something so obvious, I tried not to. If I did, it would hit me: "Wow, I'm really in prison." I would look around and say, "I'm really here. How the hell did this happen?" I was definitely not in Kansas anymore and, like Dorothy, I felt I could blunder into danger at any time. As time went on, those feelings faded.

The nonstop upheavals up the hill were part of our problem down in the camp. The administration couldn't be bothered with us small fish when they had bigger problems to deal with; they were essentially indifferent to the camp. The guy who ran the camp was just a low-level manager, not a warden, and he seemed to not want to be there. This was just another rung, and one he apparently hoped was a short one, on the prison management ladder. We never saw the warden or any of the higher-ups.

We weren't behind the walls or even fences. That lack of confinement was almost cruel. Like setting a plate of chocolate in front of a five-year-old and telling her she can't have any. Freedom is right there, but no, you can't have it. I heard that off beyond the fields there were fences, but I would've had to venture out of bounds to see them.

The interesting part was that in the place that lacked compassion, I was finding more within myself. And I tried to break up my complaining with more pleasant updates about life inside.

I am getting along well with my bunk mates. We are the only white guys on our wing and we read a lot (unlike the rest of the wing).

It's funny because we share the Wall Street Journal, as well as US magazine, so we have interesting conversations: the European Debt Crisis and Demi Moore's latest trip to rehab. We love arguing over which celebrity looked sexier wearing the same dress. Our Latino neighbors haven't quite figured us out so they now call us "SWGs"...Special White Guys! This is all done with good humor and we all joke about it. However, you will know the day I truly become institutionalized is when I start going to prison karaoke. :)

I stumbled onto a piano hidden in the chapel and was able to play a bit the past few nights. Aside from being rusty, it was great to bang the keys. I may ask Maria to send some of my sheet music. I'm hoping to take guitar lessons but am waiting for the inmates to organize and get the admin people to buy guitar strings for the 3 broken guitars. Hope this happens as I always wanted to play the guitar.

The yoga practice continues in a very positive way. While still mainly a physical practice, we have been working on breathing techniques to deal with stress "off the mat"..

One of my students has a serious anger management problem (and is receiving separate treatment for it). I met him Sunday morning for a 2-hour Power Yoga session (he's incredibly fit) and he was proud to tell me of an episode at work where he used breathing to control his temper. He attributed it to yoga and not to the other counseling. He knows this is just one step, but was encouraged by his ability to control his anger even for a short period.

Thank you all, dear friends. I wish you a happy and healthy week, and hope to be in better spirits next week.

Love & gratitude,
Mike

Bull did have anger issues, a problem he acknowledged. He was a study in contrasts. His size and demeanor had some afraid of him, but when I first met him with his words of comfort about my brother's death, he was far from intimidating.

Steve, whose opinion I respected on many things, also vouched for what a good guy Bull was, and certainly they had both welcomed me into their little circle. Most of the time Bull was very pleasant, friendly, and kind, but I had already seen flashes of anger.

I had met Bull my first day in camp, as he's part of my bunkie Steve's card group. They usually played cards two nights a week, mainly poker and hearts. They had a set group of guys and an alternate when someone couldn't make it. About five weeks into my stay, Steve invited me to join the card game (which was also where I met Rain Man). Eventually as guys left, I became a regular in the game.

Steve used to nag people—just annoying little pokes—thinking he was being funny. Bull would get angry if he lost at cards, which Steve found amusing because we weren't even playing for anything—not even fish. If Bull lost, Steve would needle him just to piss him off, jokingly calling him a loser. That first night I was invited to play, Steve was teasing Bull and Bull suddenly lost it. He threw the cards, threw his chair—it was like a scene of Bobby Knight courtside. I thought Bull was going to kill Steve and the outburst scared me. Bull stormed out of the room. I didn't know him well enough to know if I should follow him or if he'd kill me.

I suggested Steve might want to go after him and Steve, every bit as stubborn as Bull, said, "What the fuck is up with that? He needs help. He has serious anger issues." Bull clearly did have anger problems, which made me wonder why Steve, who was an otherwise good guy, provoked him.

They had overlapped in Lewisburg by about eight months at that point, so Steve knew him well enough to think he wouldn't really kill anyone. This was apparently not the first time they had had this scene together. "Where do you think he got that nickname?" Steve asked me. "He's like a fucking bull in a china shop and needs to calm down."

The next day, I saw Bull in the lunch line. On other days, I had seen him get pissed when people cut in line, steal food, or break other minor rules. I asked him about the incident at the card game and he said, "I am fucking done with that Mary and his bullshit!"

I asked him why he let Steve get to him, and that led to discussions of anger management. I suggested we work out together or that he might want to come to one of my yoga or discussion groups. I was a little surprised when he agreed. He soon became one of my closest friends at Lewisburg, which got a little awkward when a few months later Bull and Steve stopped speaking to each other; Steve even stopped coming to card games.

After the FDC, I was a little guarded in befriending people, but from the start with his condolences about my brother, there was something I liked about Bull. I grew to trust him with my fears and dreams. He was the one person I would vent to when things were not going well. Bull could often get me to laugh my way out of a funk, and I knew that attitude more than circumstances would keep me content. He had a raw sense of humor and could often get me to laugh even when I didn't think I could. When the weather got better, we would walk the track together and talk for hours.

Chapter Fourteen
Yogi Mike

Life is one long yoga flow.
We mindfully transition from one pose to another
and eventually the poses seep into our core being,
freeing us from fear and self-judgment.

Dear Friends,

Well another week has passed and happy to report things were much better this week. No headaches, no lockdowns, and no toenails on the bathroom floor... what more can one ask for? Funny how time can change our perspective on life. Last week I was so down and this week I am up, yet nothing fundamentally changed. I'm still here in prison and while the comfort level of being here has improved, there is really nothing different going on. The mood swing was not caused by changes in my circumstances; it was changed by my perception of the environment. I found myself re-reading letters of support from all of you and realized (yet again) that I am not alone here, that you are with me in spirit. This is something I'm trying to internalize because it's such a powerful force. Many of you know that I have a tendency to get into these funks where I see the world caving in on me. I suppose we all experience this feeling from time to time. Sometimes we are so self-consumed by our perception of doom and gloom that we are blind to those around us who provide us with loving support. I remain incredibly fortunate and grateful for the loving support you continue to shower me with. Many of you also know that I sometimes get caught up in details and miss the big picture. Living in the bubble world of the Lewisburg camp where compassion is a rarity, I sometimes let its negative power affect my mood and disposition. But this is just the minutiae that goes with being in prison. Your letters reflect that there is a much greater force out there, one full of love and compassion. For this I thank you for throwing me a lifeline and pulling it close to you.

The pre-GED classes continue to improve as I get more students. A lot of these guys are embarrassed that they are 40-something years old and don't have a high school diploma. They feel an obligation to tell me all the reasons why they didn't get their diploma, usually related to drugs or gangs. I tell them I'm not here to judge them and that it's my job to help them acquire the skills so they can get their degree. So far so good—obviously a good fit for me as I enjoy preparing daily lessons and interacting with the students.

One of the other pre-GED teachers had been the head of one of the largest telecommunications companies in the world, and he sometimes would get impatient with students.

A lot of his frustration stemmed from the firm belief that he didn't deserve to be there. He repeatedly told me and anyone who would listen, "These charges were completely manufactured and the verdict was set before the trial started! And it's all because I wouldn't cooperate with the government spying on people."

Some guys would tell him:

"We all got screwed, get over it."

"We each have a sob story. We don't need to hear yours."

"If anyone shouldn't be here, it's Mike. He only had a misdemeanor."

"No, my case is different," he'd protest. "The government asked me to do something illegal and I wouldn't! So they targeted me!"

He sounded like a paranoid nutcase with no interest in letting go of his righteous indignation over his case, and occasionally some of his bitterness would boil over to his students.

When he wasn't teaching, he was writing, always writing. He wanted to tell his side of things—he was spouting the sort of nonsense that I would expect from a kook wearing a tinfoil hat as he railed against government conspiracies. At this point, he had done about three years and had about two more to go, but at the rate the rage was building in him, I wasn't sure he could last that long.

His story was that the government was forcing all of the telecommunications companies to sign an agreement that they would turn over everyone's phone records and allow the government to listen in on all of the calls those companies handled. He said he refused. He told the government that they didn't have that right and would need a warrant on an individual basis for him to give up anything. He said there were veiled threats against him, but he still refused. The next thing he knew he was getting charged with all sorts of crimes. He warned us that all our private calls were being monitored, and that the government was watching us more than we could imagine.

The crazy part is, he may not have been crazy. After I was out and heard about the NSA snooping into phone records and all the revelations Edward Snowden made, I began to wonder. Everything I was reading completely backed up the story he had been trying to tell us.

Strange, the people I met in prison. Whether I had cause to complain about being in prison or not, it was where I was, and although I would vent to my friends for the most part, I did try to make the best of my time, relatively short as it was.

Yoga keeps chugging along as attendance has been increasing due to word of mouth. Taught 4 classes this weekend and will probably start a gentle yoga class for some of the elderly inmates (why are there

80+-year-old men here anyway?). Several students continue to seek more and more knowledge about the power of controlled breathing, relaxing in difficult poses, and the spiritual aspects of the practice. This has been so rewarding as it's helped deepen my practice while getting enjoyment watching other people "get it."

While there were no lockdowns this week, there was a major shakedown at one of the factories where inmates work, where they found several cell phones and synthetic marijuana. This expanded into a shakedown of a bunch of cubicles where more contraband was found. When contraband is found, they haul all the people from the cubicle into the "hole" until someone confesses. 10 people were hauled away on Wednesday with no sight of them as of Sunday night. While I could move to another cubicle with just one other bunkmate, I will remain in my 3-bunk cubicle, as I trust my bunk mates. I'm fortunate to have good bunkies and don't want to risk getting into a bad situation with a random bunk assignment.

The cell phone situation was another piece of the insanity. Some prisoners worked outside the camp, and every day they would board buses and be taken to a local factory where they disassembled cell phones and televisions for recycling. After drumming it into the men that cell phones were up there with drugs as far as contraband went, they sent prisoners to work with unlimited numbers of cell phones. When I heard this, I thought, *what the hell?* It's like sending recovering alcoholics to work in a bar.

Of course the temptation was too much for many of the guys, and they often ended up taking a phone or two or ten. Then guys would figure out a way to reactivate the phones. There was a small business of selling calls for fish. As much as I hated waiting in line for the pay phones and having others overhear my personal calls, it was not worth the risk of getting caught with a phone, which would almost certainly get me sent to the SHU and add time to my sentence.

In addition to the absurdity of letting inmates work with items they were forbidden to possess, the other thing that bothered me about this was that the BOP was getting paid several dollars per hour per prisoner and, in turn, the prisoner was paid several cents per hour.

The fact that the vast majority of the guys who worked in the factory were African American just exacerbated my feeling that this was little better than government-sanctioned slavery. How else was it legal for a private company and the BOP to be making a profit on the barely compensated labor of workers? The work buses were called "slave" buses. At times I found myself sounding like a Marxist, with my condemnation of the system and the ownership of the means of production.

I could have opted to work in the factory. Some guys liked it because it got them out of our little camp to see a slice of the world. Others found it frustrating to drive through the small city of Lewisburg and see kids going to school, people going shopping or eating at McDonald's, doing all of the mundane things that we were no longer free to do.

The BOP may have been paying me pennies an hour, fifteen cents an hour to be exact, but it was work that benefited the men I was teaching. It was work I would have done for free as a volunteer—I sure wasn't doing it for the money.

Besides being used to make calls, the illicit phones served another function—getting rid of people. Inmates were known to plant a phone in the cubicle or even the specific bunk or bin of someone they didn't like. The next inspection would turn it up and that someone got a trip to the hole. No one dared get caught snitching, but there was a box, sort of like a suggestion box, where an inmate could write a "cop out"—an anonymous tip telling the COs that someone had a phone or other contraband.

If the phone was found in a shared part of the cubicle, the cops expected the guilty party to fess up. Of course, if the phone belonged to none of them, no one would confess, and they'd all get sent to the SHU until someone cracked. But again, if no one was guilty, no one would confess, and they all might be in solitary in the Big House for a while.

There was a guy on our wing who never had money and was always trying some hustle to get some. He eventually fell deeply into debt. No one wanted to give him the beat down they thought he deserved—to get caught fighting was worse than getting caught with a phone, and anyone who was in the camp was not likely to risk a long stretch in the Big House for a violent infraction. Someone planted a phone in the debtor's bunk. I think everyone knew what happened—the cops weren't completely stupid and may have suspected it was a setup—but he never returned to camp.

I had bunkies I trusted not only to not plant things in my bunk, but to keep an eye to make sure no one else did either. There were no doors on the cubicles, so anyone could walk in or out at any time. Another thing I liked about my bunkies is they, like me, did their socializing outside of the cubicle. Other guys seemed to always have people hanging out in their cubicles. It was crowded with even just the residents, and of course the more people they had in and out, the more risk someone could take or leave something. On rare occasions, when my bunkies weren't around, I would tutor one of my students in our cubicle, but for the most part, we all went elsewhere to see our friends.

———

An amazing amount of prohibited substances made it into the camp. Because there were no fences around the camp, a visitor could hike in, stash something near the wooded part of the camp, and then a prisoner could wander out and pick it up. It was risky for both parties, but it was actually rather easy to pull off.

I could have gotten real booze from the outside or bought homemade booze. I used to watch movies and TV shows, including *Stalag 17* and *Hogan's Heroes*, about the resourcefulness of American POWs, but I thought they were exaggerated. After seeing what guys were capable of making or smuggling into the Lewisburg Camp, I had to reevaluate my opinion.

People also managed to get drugs into prison. Pills were of course easier to smuggle and hide than weed or something else that might require smoking or a syringe to get high, and lots of prescription drugs made it from the pill line to the black market. There were twice-daily pill lines, and anyone who was on meds of any sort had to queue up for the prescription. After morning count the word would be passed, "The candy man is here." The guards would watch to make sure people swallowed, but like everything else, it was a joke, and I saw many pills get smuggled out—illegal drugs were more readily available in prison than out.

Cigarettes were available on the black market, but they were expensive—sometimes a fish or two per cigarette. I guess guys with a nicotine addiction would pay whatever they had to for a fix. Smoking was completely banned, and of course it was hard to find a place to light up inside without the smell giving it away. But inmates had found many places outside to have their unofficial smoking sections. It was cheaper to share smokes and if a guard came, the men could scatter and run. The cop might catch only one or two, and it was sort of a game of musical chairs as to who might get caught with the butt in his mouth. Running too far or too fast or the wrong direction could lead to a charge of attempted escape; I had seen guys sent to the real pen with years tacked onto their sentences, all for a cigarette.

— — —

Dealing with addicts was another thing I'd have done differently if I ran this show. I knew a lot of people who had quit—or tried to quit—smoking in the real world, and they got very cranky. Forcing them to go cold turkey under what were already irritable circumstances in camp, with no support, nicotine gum or patches, or any other palliative methods, seemed to invite trouble.

Kicking a nicotine habit was one thing, but many men entered the camp (or the real prison) with serious drug addictions, and there was little to no help for them. The prison did allow people who entered with drug problems to get into a program, but only for the last year of their sentence. It meant they struggled on their own for a long time. It was hard enough to adapt to a life of incarceration, but I couldn't imagine trying to cope with a dependence on alcohol, drugs, or cigarettes at the same time.

It became obvious rather quickly that about a third of my fellow inmates needed a drug treatment center more than they needed a prison. About another third would have been better served getting treatment in a mental hospital. And about a third actually had no mental or addiction issues and made a conscious decision to do something wrong.

Sometimes there was overlap between the addicts and the criminals. I met very successful businessmen who let their addictions control their lives to the point that they ended up stealing or engaging in other criminal activity to support their habits.

Like most people who never thought they'd go to prison, I gave little thought to prison reform until I was in the system. Now I want to see it changed so that it will serve the people in prison better, which in turn will better society. Restorative justice is starting to creep into the periphery of the criminal justice system in the U.S. In places where it has been tried, it has been met with great success. After seeing the waste of money and lives in our current methods of incarceration, it is obvious from a humane or financial point of view that something needs to change. We can't keep building prisons and warehousing such a huge portion of our people. So many men I met were never taught the basics of reading and writing, let alone applicable job know-how or basic life-coping skills—how did we expect them to function in society?

While avoiding dealing with those big issues, the cops and administration kept focusing on small-time infractions, like who might be sneaking a smoke. On that score as well as many others, Lewisburg Camp often seemed more like a poorly run high school than a prison.

— — —

I tried to stay squeaky clean and not have any forbidden items in my cubicle, but the chow hall food was so disgusting, at one point I got desperate and went on the black market to buy six hardboiled eggs, paying three fish for them. I bought mayo and tortilla wraps at the commissary and was going to make egg sandwiches.

While I had the contraband eggs stashed under my mattress pad, it would be one of the few times our cubicle was singled out for a search. The guards made a lot of noise coming with their heavy boots and lots of keys jangling on chains. I am not sure if it was meant to be deliberately intimidating with the sound effects, but if that weren't enough, usually an inmate would take it upon himself to walk briskly to the bathroom, whispering a warning to each cubicle he passed.

In the few seconds of warning I had, there would be no time to re-hide the eggs. The search was often followed by a body and cavity search to make sure we had not hidden anything on our persons. The guards stopped at our cubicle and ordered us all to stand out in the aisle. The search began. They started dumping out our bins and ripping the covers off the bunks. I was sweating and trying not to lose my composure, knowing I had the illegal eggs hidden under my mattress pad. I was shitting bricks. I tried not to panic as I played out various scenarios in my head of what would happen if the cops found the eggs. I knew I would have to admit the eggs were mine and not allow my bunkies to be punished for my crime.

Technically, hiding contraband could have earned me a trip to the SHU, but it was definitely selective enforcement. I knew a trip to the hole was unlikely since I had never been in trouble before. I'd likely get a shot. Or if I was lucky, maybe they would just take the eggs and yell at me.

I saw Latinos or African Americans sent to the SHU for the most arbitrary things—having too many fish or too many stamps; some cops used any infraction as an excuse to get rid of prisoners they didn't like.

As the cops were getting to my bunk, they realized they were in the wrong cubicle. They'd had a tip about the one next door, but hit ours by mistake. They left to ransack that one. I breathed a huge sigh of relief. As soon as the coast was clear, I decided I couldn't wait to make a sandwich and risk having the eggs found in my possession. I ate two and sold the other four on the black market. I took a loss on the resale, but I just wanted them gone. After that scare, I was very careful about what I bought or hoarded.

I always felt bad when I resorted to black market food, because I knew it was food that had been stolen from the kitchen intended for the entire camp, but it was the only way to get certain things. Few eggs ever found their way to the chow line.

There were other issues around food. People cut in line all the time, especially on days when chicken was served. It was one of the few decent meals they ever had. The back third of the line probably wouldn't get any chicken and they knew it, so they tried to sneak up ahead and cut in with their friends. In the Big House, if someone cut in line they'd probably be beat up or killed, but at the camp, where no one wanted to risk the SHU for fighting, people could cut in without ramifications. It's not acceptable in the rules of common etiquette, inside prison or out, but other than some nasty looks or a few angry words, there were really no ramifications. Some cops did stop people from doing that, but infrequently. Most of the line formed up outside of the chow hall, where the guards rarely went, so it was possible to jump in line just before the door opened pretty much with impunity.

One of the little amusing things about meal time is that one of the guys who had been a big-shot lawyer refused to refer to the place we ate as "the chow hall." He always called it "the dining room." Like the British officers who insisted on dressing for tea in the jungles of Africa as their way to prevent going native and to maintain a foothold in the world they left, that was this guy's way of staying sane. I found it funny, but I can't say I thought he was crazy or wrong for doing it, if some small thing like that could help him feel normal in a place so absurd.

When I found myself getting annoyed by the irrationality of my circumstances, I tried to find a way to laugh instead, and I would share the stories with my growing reading list:

> On Thurs between classes I was watching MSNBC with Ben Bernanke testifying to congress about future Federal Reserve moves. In the same room were 2 other TVs showing a Spanish soap opera and Jerry Springer (featuring sisters who seduce their sisters' husbands). I was watching Bernanke with Rain Man, as slowly our attention moved to Jerry Springer and finally looked at each other and laughed.

Rain Man smiled and said, "Welcome to hell." Another brick in the wall to becoming institutionalized! :)

By the time I had the chance to move to another cubicle, Sarge had grown to like me well enough that he asked me to stay. Sarge had realized I wasn't a bad guy, and he stopped resenting me and trying to freeze me out. With him and many of the other white-collar criminals, I found that my background as a CEO and Wharton grad carried some weight.

But getting away from the bathroom, the phones, the noisy neighbors, and to get a lower bunk that didn't require gymnastic skills to get in and out of, made the cubicle switch worth it. Another advantage of the move was that there were only two of us in my new cubicle. The other guy, Moe, was an elderly man from Maine whom I knew and got along with. But I had only been in the new space a few days when we got a third bunkie.

The new guy, Smitty, had a huge family—about eight kids—and seemed pretty devastated at being in Lewisburg. I wondered if I had that same deer-in-the-headlights look when I got to camp. I don't think so; after the FDC, I was more relieved than terrified. I tried to show him the quirks of the phone and email systems and help him settle in.

It was interesting how quickly I became an expert in all things Lewisburg, and now was paying forward the kindness and freshman orientation Steve had given me only a few months earlier. I never became part of the standing welcome committee but did become the go-to guy for all things spiritual as well as fitness.

Often I'd be introduced as "Yogi Mike," and people would sometimes bring their new bunkies to me for help: "Hey Mike, Joe here wants to get in shape, think you could help him?" There were a lot of guys who were really obese and in terrible shape, so I would try to get them on a program they could handle. I figured it would be good practice if I ever did decide to do personal training in the real world.

I also had a reputation in the pre-GED program for being helpful and would really work with guys. "Hey, Mike, Jorge is a good guy, but he's really struggling. Do you think you could work with him?" Some of the other pre-GED and GED teachers didn't have the patience for guys who weren't getting the lessons quickly enough. As long as the student was motivated and trying his best, I would stick with it and try different ways of helping him learn until I found one that worked.

One of my students simply could not get math. He could barely read, let alone do multiplication. He wanted to be a personal trainer, so I tried to change his math problems into things related to the training. "If Sam weighs 240 pounds and wants to get down to 180 pounds, how much weight would he have to lose?" And amazingly he could even do percentages and body-mass indexes as long as the math was stated in those terms. If I just asked, "What is 240 minus 180?" he would glaze over and get lost.

After Jorge got out, I heard from him a few times and he was really struggling. He loved being a personal trainer, but was barely making better than minimum wage. He was used to making six figures as a drug dealer and couldn't understand how anyone could pay rent and feed a family on the little money he was now making. I wished I had spent more time teaching him how to do a personal budget, but he was right—most families that lived within the law struggled, and I couldn't help him with that.

When I did personal training, I didn't charge. Other guys made a few fish on the side doing it. One day I was training Bull and one of the for-pay trainers was hogging most of the equipment. Bull said something to him, and in a flash they were ready to throw down. I jumped between them.

I pushed Bull away and said, "Time in the SHU? For what?"

"But someone ought to kick that little asshole's..."

"Someday someone probably will. But not you. Not here. Not now. Let it go." After that brief moment when his body kicked into survival fight-or-flight mode (and I never knew Bull to run away from anything), he, in fact, did let it go. The moment passed just as we had talked about so many times, only now it wasn't theory but real life. I told him that all of the yoga and meditations we were doing were useless if he couldn't put it into practice here and now.

We could all have gotten in trouble if a cop had seen it, so I wanted to defuse things as quickly as possible, but ultimately Bull controlled his own destiny, and I was so proud of his commitment to personal growth.

I liked Bull's passion for life. He was a big man and he lived life big. He had a wonderful sense of humor and he could be funny as hell. He also had a very serious and introspective side. He would read the books I loaned him, and he'd lend me books and we'd discuss literally anything from philosophy to religion, sports, and spousal relationships. Often we'd talk about ways to handle life's stressors without first getting angry. He, like many others in Lewisburg, was always on edge; they reached their flashpoints rather quickly and wanted to punch some of the COs or other inmates who may have very much deserved it. Everyone got worn thin by the lack of sleep and too little privacy, and it was easy to get on each other's nerves. Bull was one of the men who used his time to get to know himself—both the good and the bad—and was committed to working on finding peace within himself. I admired his commitment to "do the work."

— — —

It wasn't always easy to remain calm. Doing yoga in Lewisburg was always a challenge. The only place we were allowed to do it was in the gym. This meant weights clanking, guys grunting and yelling, and during ping-pong matches, occasionally a ball hitting someone. I tried to keep my class focused and remind them that true yoga is not the movements; yoga done right is a mental discipline. Perhaps paradoxically the chaos of the gym resulted in deeply intense and moving yoga practices. Ultimately, this paved the road toward starting group meditation classes, but I would have to find a quieter location to meditate. Later, we would find a calm place in the chapel, into which I had been sneaking to play the piano.

Been playing the piano a few times a week and find so many similarities to yoga. It's de-stressing, you can practice by yourself or in a community, you get the best results when you relax the mind and body and let the music flow through you rather than being mechanical. I was playing alone when a Latino guy came into the Chapel and asked if he could join in and play the bongos...Yes, of course. Then 2 of his friends came in and started with the congas and shakers. It was a beautiful thing—an impromptu gathering of improvised salsa music (thank God I know one salsa riff!). One of the highlight experiences so far. A neat sense of community in an otherwise awful place. BTW, the chapel has a few instruments used by the many religious groups here including Native Americans, Jehovah's Witnesses, Muslims, Amish, Rastafarians, etc. Also had opportunity to play with a guy from Pakistan, Sayed, who writes and sings beautiful Pakistani love songs. He has an amazing voice. Am fortunate to have both yoga and music available. Speaking of music...I start guitar lessons on Tuesday.

Supposedly, there was a rule about not playing the piano in the chapel unsupervised. A few cops would tell me to stop, but most didn't care. At times I would question the wisdom of this—I was risking a shot just to play the piano. I guess I couldn't fault the guys who risked a shot for a drag on a cigarette; they had their addiction and I had mine. Music helped me feel human in a place where almost everything seemed designed to strip us all of our humanity.

Like risking a shot for the taste of a decent French fry, in retrospect it was dumb. Some nights I'd lie in bed and wonder why I had risked it just to play the piano, but I guess if I had two addictions, they were piano and yoga. I guess I was fortunate that to some degree I could indulge in both of those things, unlike the guys who needed a fix of something much harder to come by in prison.

One night I was playing the piano, and a guard came in and asked what I thought I was doing. I got nervous, thinking this would be the time I was busted for sure. Instead he grabbed a guitar and asked if he could sit in. One more case of random enforcement of the rules and another glimpse of the human side of at least one of the cops.

Chapter Fifteen
Pawn Sacrifice

In society, there is a fine line between
being accepted and rejected,
thus my desire to focus on neither
and be true to myself.

I tried to keep my support team updated on all of the other aspects of my journey through the prison system. I think most people have a weird voyeurism about what life is really like in prison (but don't want to have to go there to find out), so I think some of my friends were following my tale as their vicarious inside look.

I hesitate to share the following with you as I don't want to jinx my chances, but there is a possibility that I could be released to a halfway house or home confinement at the end of July. While not a huge deal, it would mean I'd be out of here one month early. The paperwork was submitted, but I won't hear anything for about 3 months (this is the government). All of this is conditioned on having a job lined up now. Fortunately, Denise agreed to hire me back at her fitness club to teach some classes and help in some admin areas.

Friday night has become card night and we rotate who brings the food. Usually it's just something simple from the commissary like pretzels, chips or cookies. But Friday we had a feast; and Bull made pork stuffed strombolis, cheese and crackers with jalapenos and olives ... by far the best food since being sentenced. He acquired the ingredients through the underground market; cooked them on an iron and wrapped them in a metal material used on the outside rolls of building insulation. Let's hope he cleaned all the asbestos off. He even built a pizza delivery box to transport food from his cubicle to the card room. My turn is next week, but no way to match this!!!

I was in awe of what Bull could create seemingly out of nothing. With the limited resources of the commissary, what he could scrounge from the chow hall, and only a steam iron on which to cook, he could conjure up meals that even given Martha Stewart's kitchen, I couldn't have reproduced. Sometimes he'd explain, "I didn't have any A so I substituted B. I didn't have any Y so I substituted Z." He was a MacGyver of food who could make a recipe that was three-quarters replacement ingredients and have it come out delicious. Occasional angry outbursts aside, it was a treat to have him in our card group. I always felt bad that I could never come close to matching his culinary skills, but I also knew he took pride in being in a cooking league of his own. Bull was a host of contradictions. He was the kind of guy who would be scary to meet in a bar and could be quick tempered, but he also had a gentle side and had the patience to painstakingly create fabulous meals for his friends.

We had many long talks about our paths, the mistakes he had made, and how it pained him that his father seemed unwilling to ever forgive him. He feared his father would die before they ever made peace. I knew the yoga and discussion groups were working with Bull, and I tried to expand those programs to help others.

Dear Friends,

Things here are good, as I've been busy with many activities...maybe too busy. I've been describing the development of a yoga program here...generally with positive results. More importantly, participants are embracing the asanas (poses) and have been open to other aspects of yoga including mindfulness, anger management, keeping positive, breathing, etc.

I've been gradually adding elements of breathing, meditation, and self-reflection to the yoga sessions. The inmates are taking this on with positive outcomes in their overall well-being.

Given the desire to go deeper, we approached the chaplain (who is also a correctional officer) to allow us to use the chapel on off hours. The gym is just too noisy for meditation and the chapel is about the only quiet spot on the compound. We received a scathing reply denying the request saying that we shouldn't be polluting inmates with this stuff as inmates will get confused into believing that yoga is a religion and that these programs cannot be part of the Bureau of Prisons. Very frustrating and very tempting to throw up your hands and just give up.

Fortunately my students "get it" so we will try to find another way (I'm thinking of sneaking into the rec room where guitar lessons are taught).

The food situation has reached an all-time low and I skipped dinner when they served 'sewer trout' (some kind of tuna fish that was literally inedible) and made a spam sandwich in my cubicle. I used 2 slices of stale bread (which I saved from dinner 2 nights ago) and a package of spam which I bought from the commissary. I used margarine spread in lieu of mustard and washed it down with a carton of milk (saved from breakfast). Either my taste buds have been burned out or they changed the taste of spam as I really enjoyed the sandwich.

Was thinking they should make a TV show of this place kind of like M*A*S*H as it's a similar environment where you have periods of nothing, watching goofy things happen. Then there are periods of intensity watching cops intimidate people. Here are a few stories: Presidents' Day Bingo was cancelled due to the lack of budget to pay for prizes...mind you the prize was a 6 pack of Hawaiian Punch (cost of $2.50) yet they just bought 3 new pickup trucks at a cost of $100,000. Also there is a debate over allowing Maxim magazine into the prison...which it has for years. Apparently a committee of cops was formed to determine if this is considered inappropriate. Personally I think the cops just want an excuse to look at the girly pictures. Last Friday I worked the Mock Job Fair where 8 outside companies came to interview inmates who have been participating in our Employment Workshop (which was a big success). The cops gave us only 1 instruction...do not look at the women in a suggestive way and avoid making eye contact with them.

I became aware that no one really runs the prison. Guards think they do, the warden thinks he does. As oppressive as the camp seemed at times, on some larger level it seemed that no one really cared. We just weren't worth worrying about compared to the killings and gang wars up the hill.

At the camp, as long as the inmates were kept reasonably under control the administration was happy. Some prisoners tried to pretend they ran the camp, and I just stayed out of their way to do my own thing.

It was a challenge finding the right path in prison. If I followed the rules too closely, tried too hard to fit in, tried to adapt too much,

I risked being robbed of myself and becoming institutionalized, something I swore I would not let happen. If I fought it too much, I could become angry and bitter or withdrawn and depressed. Some of the white-collar guys were trying so hard to feel superior while being in this place with people they thought were "beneath" them that it paved their own painful road. Even after just a few months, I could find myself slipping into a pattern and a way of being that made it difficult to remember what life was like without a strict schedule and a million petty rules. It was a fine line to walk—adapting and obeying without giving in to this as my way of life.

As I got to know many of the men better and became the confidante of many, I learned that most were embarrassed that they let their families down and let themselves down by committing crimes and ending up in prison. I am sure there were many who didn't feel that way, but then those guys weren't coming to me for advice or counsel.

As with teaching yoga, it was hard to tell sometimes if I was doing things for me that just happened to benefit other people, or if I was doing things for other people that as a side effect made me feel better.

I had learned from my experience with Bob that if I saw myself as *helping* someone else, it would skew our relationship. I was placing myself above them to stoop to raise them up to my level. If I viewed what I was doing as serving them, we were equals and I would treat them accordingly. The relationship changed to one of mutual respect.

One of the most interesting lessons for me was the relative nature of time. Here, where everything was so controlled, time was one of the least-defined things. In the outside world, when my time was supposedly my own, I was always obligated to be somewhere, doing something at all times. In Lewisburg there was an unlimited amount of time, and how we spent each minute (with several very firm scheduled events during the day—counts) was almost entirely up to us.

There were guys who did nothing all day. For me and most of the guys I chose to hang out with, we sought to pack as much as possible into each twenty-four-hour day. I felt as though I was accomplishing a lot, and it passed the time faster than staring at the walls.

Dear Friends,

Happy Wednesday and leap year. While I'm not happy to have this extra day it does mean that March is here. Few people here count the days and weeks but everyone counts the months. So with the end of February, we briefly pause to appreciate that we're one month closer to freedom.

I keep thinking that I'll run out of material to write about but so far the goofy stories keep on flowing. "Where to start...I mailed a letter using a "forever" stamp, the kind that you can use regardless if the rate goes up. As you know the postal rate increased a couple of weeks ago but this should not have been a problem except that one of the correctional officers came to my cubicle to return the letter saying I needed more postage. He didn't or couldn't understand the "forever" stamp concept and refused to take the letter until I added another stamp. After he left and I looked at my bunk mates and said, "Did this really just happen? Seriously?"

Then there's the chess game that erupted into a full-fledged fight. Never considered chess a contact sport but reality changes when you're in prison. Apparently someone moved out of turn and captured a queen then all hell broke loose. Kind of reminded me of those real-life chess games at those Renaissance Fairs only here they weren't acting. Fortunately no guards were around so no one got put into the hole. Think I'll stick with yoga as it's a lot safer :) Then there's the ongoing food saga...Sunday night is usually "sh*t on a shingle" night

(I think the c.o.'s call it beef stroganoff but it's not even close) and tastes as bad as it looks so I've become adept at cubicle cuisine and my own recipe for prison style egg salad. I've become a hoarder of usable food and am learning how to cook with an iron...kind of feel like MacGyver.

One of the pre-GED students, a 54-year-old guy, was proudly telling us he's now a great-grandfather. Yes, a great-grandfather! I did the math and it's definitely possible and he said he knows a bunch of great-grandfathers who are younger than him. Wow.

Last week a 78-year-old man started his 4-year sentence. He's very frail and has no idea how to use this crazy email and phone system. I've helped him set up his contact list. Why would you put this man in prison? Did I tell you he uses a walker? I don't know his crime but it seems cruel. He's a frightened man. Seems to me there must be a better way for him to pay his debt to society.

Finally an inmate arrived from Malvern (town next to West Chester) who was a member of the fitness center where I taught yoga. I taught him & his family yoga on Sat. afternoons. Small world.

In my last write-up I complained that I have too much on my plate and wanted to cut back...well, I did the opposite. I signed up for a self-study course to become a certified personal trainer. While I still plan to complete the more intensive program that Maria is about to graduate from, the prison program will allow me to train at a bunch of places once I get out. This is something I really want to do especially being here and working out with other inmates, as I have learned a lot just by hanging with these "muscle heads."

Unfortunately the piano playing has come to a grinding halt thanks to Fr. Pat (my favorite priest--not) who told another inmate that only religious music can be played in the chapel even during off hours. There's another broken piano in the chapel that I'd like to move to the rec room and find an inmate to repair it. I will approach the chaplain (not Fr. Pat) to see if this is possible. I will also have to get approval from the rec cop to do this so the chances are slim to none. But it sure was fun playing these past 2 weeks. Fr. Pat certainly doesn't present the Catholic Church with a compassionate face.

Bull has been reading The Four Agreements. I am grateful that Bull has taken an interest in these principles as it helps remind me to try to live by these actions. We are using the 4 Agreements to supplement his yoga practice. It's so powerful and he's seeing tremendous gains physically and emotionally.

I was happy with the way Bull was embracing all that I had to offer him in the gym, on the mat, and in mindfulness off the mat. It was my pleasure to serve as his guide for part of his journey. It has often been said that to really learn something, it is necessary to teach it. I internalized so many of the lessons I wanted to learn by sharing them with Bull. I would have some of my own best insights and moments of clarity after a long talk with Bull. In return, Bull called me out on my need for certainty, control, and order. He helped me loosen up, to not always see everything as a lesson and to explore life near the edges. One of the other things I had in common with Bull was that he had been raised Catholic and was also questioning the church's teachings, especially as embodied by Father Pat.

And I continued to report to my readers:

Greetings. Another week down and nice to have an additional hour of sunlight. The weather has been relatively mild all winter and we can feel spring around the corner. The clocks turned forward last night and already people are betting how long it takes for the COs to actually change the clocks. Odds are 4 to 1 that they will stay out of whack until it's time to turn them back in the fall! I sometimes feel like Garrison Keillor from the PBS radio show Lake Woebegone only the stories here are real and are as bizarre as ever. Here we go...

Three weeks ago, the commissary added Raisin Bran cereal to its offering. I was happy to have an alternative to grits, which has been a staple for breakfast.

We just found out that Raisin Bran along with Pop Tarts, jelly, trail mix (among others) were discontinued due to the potential of making hooch out of the raisins or jelly. Apparently this was done throughout the entire prison system. I can't even imagine drinking hooch made out of Pop Tarts or raisins.

Predictably I was unsuccessful in getting approval to use the piano or move the broken one to the rec room, however I wasn't prepared for the reason why. Apparently inmates steal piano strings to use as an instrument to make tattoos (or as we call it "getting ink"). This is the reason why it's almost impossible to get a replacement guitar string when they break. I am still so naive about prison life.

Speaking of guitars... my teacher is a tough former gang member from Maine who was busted on multiple gun and drug charges.

He's a heavy metal enthusiast, which is reflected in his teaching style and as a result I'm learning to play Metallica songs... a far cry from my smooth jazz days. There were 4 students in my group and he's already scared away 2 of them, but I'm determined to stick it out.

Yesterday I completed CPR training/certification. The training was excellent but halfway through the class 4 COs came to lecture us on prison policy that inmates are forbidden to give CPR to anyone. In fact we had to sign a form reflecting this and that we will be punished if caught trying to save someone's life. Someone asked, "then why do you offer this training?" to which the response was "to make you feel good about yourselves." Behind one of the housing units is a lovely little farm house sitting next to a barren cornfield. This house is actually a SWAT training center. Part of their training includes hassling inmates. Last week while one of the prison buses was transporting 40 inmates back to the compound after work, the SWAT guys stormed the bus brandishing guns in a mock hostage situation (I can only assume their guns were not loaded). Fortunately I was not on the bus but there were a lot of scared and angry inmates.

I continue to enjoy the 2 courses but had to t̲... ..
step back and laugh during last weeks' "New Business
Start Up" course. We had a heated debate about risk,
return, cost of capital, funding, etc. which are relevant
factors to be considered. However, what was funny
was that the debate included 2 mobsters, a former
mayor (who took bribes), 2 former gang members (guns
& drugs) and a financial guy (insider trading). Quite a
cast of characters.

I will leave you with this thought/poem which I
received from 2 people within the past 2 weeks: "Peace"
(author unknown):

It does not mean to be in a place where there is no noise,
trouble or hard work.

It means to be in the midst of those things and still be
calm in your heart.

This is something that we all strive for in the midst of
the insanity of our world today.

Chapter Sixteen
Surrender Doesn't Mean Giving Up

Acknowledge your situation and surrender to the truth.
Truth gives you the power to shed the burdens, fears, and
misconceptions that hold you back from living an authentic life.

Dear Friends:

Greetings. Four months have now passed, which means I'm 44% done with my sentence. Sure wish I was further along, but I'm almost to the halfway point. It's been another up and down week.

While life continues in here, so do the stories...so here are some highlights—or lowlights, depending on your perspective:

Students from Susquehanna Univ. (sophomore ethics class) came to the prison to see the caged animals. I know their intention was to try to "scare straight" these young students, but it was humiliating to many inmates. Students stared and pointed at us like we were animals in a zoo. At least they could have thrown us a few peanuts! Of course the COs were telling them about all the wonderful rehabilitation programs available to help turn our lives around. I think the students believed all of the BS. Personally, I don't mind the students visiting, but I don't like the distorted picture the COs present to them...probably the same type of thing goes on in North Korea. :)

There was trouble in another housing unit. Fortunately, it wasn't on my wing. They brought in alcohol. There were several guys drunk at the stand-up count. One was so drunk he couldn't walk on his own. He won't be back.

Saturday night I watched a CO use a metal detector (the kind you see on the beach) to scan the sand volleyball court, and they found two cell phones wrapped in plastic.

My bunkie, the older guy from Maine, still can't believe I'm here for a misdemeanor. He says I should kick someone's ass so I can move up to a felony.

As promised, following is a brief review of the books I've read since getting to Lewisburg.

1. Radical Acceptance, Tara Brach, PhD. Clear practical and caring guide that shows how to move shame and self-hatred to a higher level of consciousness, for loving ourselves for who we are and the incredible capacity of the human heart. Excellent introduction in basic principles of mindfulness in a clear and practical way. Good book for people interested in dealing with anxieties. Book well written in a narrative form from the author's personal experiences and her work as a clinical psychologist.

2. Living Buddha, Living Christ, Thich Nhat Hanh. This book states about as clearly as possible my belief system. It takes many aspects of Christianity and compares them to Buddhist principles. It's amazing that at a 30,000-ft. level, there are so many similarities. Thich Nhat Hahn does an amazing job of comparing the two and finding the common thread that connects all of us. I have read many of his writings and feel a strong connection to him.

3. Dr. Seuss & Philosophy – Oh, the Thinks You Can Think, Jacob Held. A series of interesting and fun essays delving into the deeper philosophical meaning behind Dr. Seuss's stories. Found it fascinating to see how deep some of his poems were.

About this time, Larry took over from Jenny as my conduit to the outside world. After months of being supportive and trying to keep things together, Jenny and I had a long talk. I knew it would be unfair of me to let her believe there was any hope of us getting back together, and she said it would be too painful for her to visit me any longer. We had been separated before my sentencing, and we agreed to separate again.

I knew this was going to be awkward and painful for my many friends, and I felt bad about hurting them—still the "pleaser" in me thinking I had let them down—but I was surprisingly at peace with the decision. I knew that more than a few guys had their marriages fall apart because of their incarceration. I would see guys on the phone or in visitation pleading with their wives to wait to file the divorce papers until after they were released to try to work things out. Other guys were given ultimatums—unless they got over their addiction, or completed their sentence and found a job or some other condition, there was no way their spouses would take them back. In a few cases, I provided an ear and support system for guys who feared they were no longer part of their own families.

In my case, my being sent away had nothing to do with my marriage falling apart. It became the final break in a rope that had been fraying for too long. Those on my reading list knew what was going on, so I stuck to more mundane topics, including the weather.

The weather has turned cold again, but the heat in the housing units was turned off several weeks ago, so we've been freezing at night. We only have two light blankets so have been sleeping in sweat pants, sweat shirt, socks and wool cap. We live in an uninsulated cement block building. I actually slept with my coat on. The cops have been disciplining people who sleep with their hats on. They bang their flashlights on our bunks to wake us up and yell at us to pull the covers off our heads. Their reasoning is that they must see our heads to insure we are alive and physically in our bunks (i.e. not a stuffed dummy there while the inmate escapes). My saga of seeking a good night of sleep continues. For the life of me, I can't understand why they treat us this way. This seems way beyond the punishment handed down by the judge. As you can imagine, this is not conducive to restful sleep. Dreaming of the day when I can sleep in peace. Poor Mr. Green, who's almost 80 years old, had to be moved to the boiler room at 3 a.m. to get some warmth.

The excuse was that the heaters were on seasonal timers, and once they were turned off for the year, that was it until winter. In other words, the heat was controlled by the calendar, not the thermostat. In the night, sometimes you couldn't help instinctively putting your head under the covers to stay warm, and some cops would actually write shots to prisoners who did this. I somehow never got a shot, but as bad as it was to be awakened so they could shine a flashlight in my face, I can't imagine how much more aggravating it would be to have to stand up and be written up for this.

Instead of being angry, I would try to remember my mantra: *Joy. Surrender. True self.*

And not only practicing yoga, but at this point, more importantly, sharing it did bring joy and the right kind of surrender.

The yoga program continues nicely. The students and program progress, and I find it rewarding to see the guys take to it. Part of the discipline of the practice is to stay calm and focused in the face of distraction and discomfort. Boy, there are many opportunities to practice here. Yesterday we practiced next to two ping pong tables during a tournament with balls flying all over the place... some hitting us during Warrior I and Tripod pose. Rather than getting frustrated, we used this as a learning opportunity to stay focused, control our breath, to be aware of our surroundings, but not to let it overwhelm us. I think the prison experience will significantly change my approach to teaching when I get back on the streets.

We were finally approved to set up a meditation program. I met a new inmate who is Hindu and interested in meditation. He was approved by the chaplain for meditation. I'm very excited about this and we have several experienced meditation guides to lead us through different techniques. I will lead the yoga nidra practice. The first session will start Monday night. Meditation will be an awesome supplement to the yoga practice.

Again there was the conundrum of whether yoga was a religion. If we left out the "yoga" part, we could call it meditation and use the chapel. We still did the asanas in the gym, but the relative quiet of the chapel was nice for the "nidra" part. One hour a week wasn't really enough, and soon another guy came to camp who said he was a Buddhist. I got him to request the chapel for an hour for Buddhist time. Funny, but the Buddhist time looked a lot like the Hindu time that looked a lot like yoga nidra. I felt a little sneaky essentially lying—not exactly lying, but bending the truth a tad. It was one of those cases where the end seemed to justify the means. If the prison administration had been reasonable, we wouldn't have had to resort to this.

We did half an hour of yoga nidra followed by another half an hour of optional men's discussion group. I wasn't sure how many would stick around for that, but no one left, and it became an integral and helpful part of the entire mindfulness practice I was slowly building.

— — —

The title "yogi" is a sign of respect. Not every yoga practitioner or instructor is a yogi; a yogi is someone who really gets the teachings and walks the walk. I had met so many yoga teachers who wanted to call themselves yogis, but off the mat they were horrible people. They wanted to wear the clothes, and pose on the mat, but when it came to actually helping people, forget it—it was all about them, not the students.

In prison I found several "seekers" who were on similar paths—trying to learn more about themselves and the universe. I had learned different philosophies, and with my spiritual awakening I tried to share those ideas with others without sounding like a know-it-all or a guru. I wasn't some mystic; I was a business guy who stumbled upon yoga and found it helpful. After years of wandering—feeling lost, but not knowing how or why or even how to tell anyone I was, I felt I was where I was supposed to be and helping others to find their own paths.

Many of the guys told me that they saw me as a rock, a place of calm behind which they could find safe harbor. I was not a saint and certainly not immune from doubts and dark moments, but my mini-breakdowns were few and not severe. There were, however, many sleepless nights and doubting days that I tried to keep to myself.

I felt worst when I thought about the burden placed on my family and friends. That was a common problem for the guys inside—feeling awful and guilty about how they had disappointed their loved ones on the outside. I had some of those feelings, but since my crime was very different, I didn't have quite the same type of guilt and felt less of a disappointment to my family.

My family and friends also provided me so much support and strength and never acted as though I were burdening them. They were there for visits, phone calls, books, and gifts. I felt extremely fortunate and had enough support and caring that I could share with my friends and followers in the camp. My brother Larry came almost every weekend when visitations were allowed. My younger brother Brendan came when he could, and brought my dad once. Distance kept my sister Mary from visiting often, but she was my number one source of letters and books. She and I had very similar tastes in reading material, so if she read a book and liked it, she would send me a copy. In the times that I felt myself getting down or feeling lonely, I'd try to remember the awesome group I had propping me up.

So many guys would get calls or visits from their families in which, instead of being greeted with love and support, they were met with anger, resentment, and guilt.

Rather quickly, I had developed a sort of Zen approach about everything in prison. Pushing too hard, being too anxious, and wanting time to pass quickly was likely to end in frustration. The best thing that I, and others who had learned to cope, found to do was just accept it. It was what it was. In yoga, we frequently use the term "surrender." To me, surrendering doesn't mean giving up. It means making the best of your situation. I was in prison and I couldn't change this reality, yet I could release the anger and the frustration of why I was in prison and be present to the experience of life.

An inmate approached me to talk about yoga off the mat and we got into a deep discussion about how we need to use this time to improve ourselves. He's from Coatesville (very near West Chester), 32 years old, and been in prison since he was 22. This guy is amazing, as he's completely turned his life around. He's in incredible physical shape and has the respect of all the inmates. We're planning to keep in touch and maybe find a non-profit project to work together on. Meeting people like him helps offset the craziness of being here.

Chapter Seventeen
Earning a PhD in Self

Underneath the masks we wear, people are people.
We all come from different life circumstances and have made
decisions that have affected the quality of our lives,
yet there is a core life force that connects us.

Another week or so has passed. I hope you all had a nice Easter. As previously noted, the holidays are generally quiet here. Holidays are generally not good occasions here and I'm happy to only have two holidays left: Memorial Day and July 4th.

My brother Brendan was kind enough to bring my father for a visit. It was great seeing him along with Erin and Maria.

I joined a softball team despite my intention not to (due to the potential for injury and relying on medical treatment here). However I will be playing in the "B" league, which is less competitive, and will be playing with my buddies. I need to work on saying "no"! I will also be playing in a bocce league. I've never played bocce before but it looks like shuffle board played on grass. My teammate is Rain Man, who has also never played. I have low expectations for performance, but high expectations for fun. Anything to make the time go by!

One of my friends who hadn't seen me in months and finally made it to visit commented on how ripped I was getting. Indeed, with all the time in the world to work out and not much food to eat, it is relatively easy to get in shape, although I wouldn't recommend getting locked away as the best way to start a fitness program. The gym was crowded and filthy, but there were weights and Nautilus machines held together with duct tape and other makeshift repairs, but from what I'd heard, other prisons didn't even have that much—certainly the FDC didn't— so I was grateful to have this much to work with.

We will need a larger room for meditation—there is such a pent up need. What's been so neat is that meditation crosses race, religion, and all socio-economic factors. After meditation class, an impromptu discussion session formed where people opened up about their goals in life, how they are coping with prison, how to prepare for the disgrace of returning to the outside world and the impact on their personal life (failed marriages, etc.). Pretty powerful stuff which spontaneously morphed after meditation. I've been taken back by the popularity of this program, all of which is being done below the radar screen with no support from admin. Imagine what we could accomplish if prison admin would recognize the benefits of meditation...but I won't get on my soap box this week.

Our Saturday night card games have morphed into food cuisine challenges as we rotate trying to make new and tasty appetizers. Last week we had pizzas with olives, freeze dried habanera beans, turkey sausage, and cheese. This was served with a "house" dip consisting of squeeze cheddar cheese, smushed mackerel, Thai hot sauce, and refried beans, served on saltine crackers. One of the guys concocted a new frozen coffee drink called a "con-uccino" (a poor man's cappuccino), made with instant coffee, hot chocolate mix, powdered vanilla creamer, sugar, and water. It's always an experience and the card game is secondary. I previously mentioned that an elderly gentleman, John, joined the group, and he's now affectionately known as "Papa John."

Not many humorous stories to relate, but here are a couple...

1. The new correctional officer caught an inmate with a cell phone and chased him when he took off. He ended up tearing his Achilles heel and is out for 30 days. The CO only caught a glimpse of the inmate's backside, so has been checking out inmates' butts to see if he can find a match!

2. Where else but in prison can you find 2 CEOs, 2 drug dealers, and a mortgage fraud guy playing the board game Risk? That's what they were doing at the table next to our card game last night. What a place!

3. One of my new students recently transferred in from a camp in Texas, where his GED teacher was the (infamous) guy who sent fake anthrax packages to a bunch of U.S. Senators back in 2001. He received a 15-year sentence, but apparently is an excellent teacher!

4. Funny story during one of my solo yoga sessions. I was briefly resting on my stomach in between "bow" poses in the back corner of the gym, when an inmate comes over and shakes me. He thought I was unconscious and wanted to give me CPR! He recently got his CPR certification and was all excited to try it out. He immediately apologized and we both laughed about it. I use these events as ways to deepen my practice.

All in all not such a bad time here. For someone used to travelling all over the place, it has been a struggle to keep sane living in the 15-acre compound. While I continue to miss the little things from the outside world (like Dunkin Donuts coffee, food, heat) there are many moments of levity and things to be thankful for. I continue to make the best of a bad situation, as the alternative is not so attractive.

Each inmate was supposed to be present for mail call, and I got a lot of letters and books. I felt bad, because some guys were waiting for weeks for one letter. They would show up every day and wait for their name to be called and it never would be. Meanwhile, I'd get something every day. As I got busier, I paid someone to get my mail. Most guards knew what was up and didn't care, but every once in a while, the guy getting my mail and I would both get in trouble for that. Because I got so much mail, when I did show up, the guard who usually did mail call knew my name and would ask how I was doing. It was odd to see such flashes of humanity from most of the cops at the camp, but it was nice. Late in my sentence, that cop asked if I was out of there soon. Again it took me by surprise to have any CO express what seemed to be genuine concern or interest. Sometimes I wrote snail mail replies to the many letters I got, but most of the time I wrote general missives that would be shared with my friends.

Thought for the day... patience.

Being here forces a degree of patience, whether it be watching people cut in line for chow, waiting for a computer terminal to free up, being sent back to our cubicle in the middle of yoga for "emergency counts," waiting in line for commissary only to find they are out of stock on the stuff you really wanted, having no lights in the bathroom for 3 days (bulbs burned out and took 3 days for them to be replaced) ... Well, the list goes on but you get the point. Patience is the key to survival and it is difficult for many of the Type-A white-collar guys.

This place provides the opportunity to observe peoples' behavior and our reaction to it. Patience is valuable when teaching students who, despite their best efforts, can't grasp basic concepts in math and reading. I'm hoping that a stronger sense of patience will follow me onto the street as I can see where I could have used a lot more patience in my personal life.

My daughter once described me as the most Type-A yogi she had ever seen, and she may have been right. Now I was learning patience. Again, when the student is ready, the teacher will appear. The teacher of patience was the thousand inconveniences of life as a guest of the BOP.

The other activities continue on with softball starting this week. We've had two practices so far. I haven't played softball in about 20 years, so lots of cobwebs to clean out. I'll be playing first base, the position I played in high school. Our team name is The Nationals—which, if we play like the real Nationals, our prospects aren't so good.

Sometimes I believe I'm living in an alternate reality with the stuff that goes on here. I think it's a sign of the apocalypse when you have several 65-year-old white-collar guys singing songs by LMFAO including Party Rock (they especially love to sing that part "everyday I'm shuffling") along with the young, physically fit black guys singing "Rumor Has It" by Adele. If I wasn't in prison, I'd think this was hysterical! The big news here is that the commissary started selling the new M&M's chocolate covered pretzels. They are tasty but not as good as the hype. They shut off the TVs in the other housing unit for a week as punishment for someone pooping on the floor by the phones in the common area. Pretty disgusting, but we think it may have been done by poor Mr. Green (the 80 year old), who has a long list of medical problems.

A white-collar guy self-surrendered to camp a month ago. After 5 days here, he was sent to the hole for 15 days due to insubordination...He missed the daily count (which he said he didn't know about since he was new) and didn't respond to his name being paged over the PA system. The CO said he needed an "attitude adjustment" thus the trip to the hole. I met the guy yesterday (he's an incredibly talented guitar player), who explained the entire ordeal (at least his side of the story). It really doesn't matter who you were on the outside, as we are all the same inside—a good lesson about letting go of the ego.

I had to ask myself why I was willing to risk injury playing ball in a place where medical care ranged from nonexistent to poor, but I guess with the coming of spring, I was a little restless and stir crazy. And I had to admit, I wanted to reconnect with baseball. Since high school, I had slowly drifted away from my first childhood passion. Here in this artificial environment was a chance to give it another try. No one in my real life would have to know if I made a fool of myself.

I always told myself I wasn't *that* old and I could still play. In the last three decades, I had held a bat only a few times. While I was at Synthes, we played a few of the low-pressure fun games of typical picnic-style softball and I could still hit okay. I used to be a power hitter in high school—batting fifth in the line-up, sort of second cleanup behind our cleanup hitter, who was really good and had been drafted by some pro teams right out of high school.

I loved baseball, but after choosing not to even try out for the college team, then raising two girls who couldn't care less about the sport, I stopped paying attention to it other than an occasional trip to a Phillies game as more of a social outing. Maria particularly hated baseball, so if I wanted time with her—and as much as I traveled, I did—I wouldn't waste hours in front of the TV to watch a game. So I pretty much lost all interest in baseball, and Lewisburg would be a chance to reconnect with that part of my youth.

But at Lewisburg, where the teams seemed to take this way too seriously given the ludicrous setting, a strange thing happened. I couldn't hit at all. They played slow-pitch with the super-high arc, and it was hard to get my timing down to hit anything.

Of course that subjected me to the jeers of the other players— both the opposing team and my own bench. I wasn't sure which the bigger objective of these games and practices was: to score the most runs or the most jabs at anyone who messed up. The ribbing and taunting were merciless.

After a few frustrating at-bats, I decided to bring the calm of yoga to the batter's box. I would breathe. Just as I had learned to tune out the grunting of the weightlifters in the gym, I would tune out the heckling. I would just be in the moment, watching the ball. I would wait and I would accept the outcome—a hit or a miss—as equally okay and be at peace with that. It was a far different approach to the game than I'd had at Christian Brothers Academy.

And it worked. I started hitting. For power. I brought in a few game-winning runs before the season was over. I was so relaxed on the diamond that it was here that the nickname "Yogi Mike" really took hold. And when the teasing crossed the line and guys threatened to make the taunts physical, I was often asked to step in and calm things down. The crazy nature of these games was that altercations were as likely to break out among teammates as between opposing benches.

Fernando, who had first dubbed me and my cubicle mates "Special White Guys" also wanted to play softball. He was only about 5'8" but very bulky and muscular, and he couldn't play baseball. He was awkward and uncoordinated, but he had trusted me to tutor him toward his GED, and after seeing how I turned around my hitting, he asked me to tutor him with his. Amazingly, he managed to prove himself at the plate.

Of all the little victories at Lewisburg, this was one of the most rewarding. I rekindled my love for the sport and was able to share it with someone. I loved that I could apply yoga to my first love, baseball, with good results.

After I got out, I didn't feel any desire to find a men's softball league. I'd had my fun and sort of proved my theory that yoga could provide benefits well off the mat—all the way to home plate. Now my family and I go to a couple of Phillies games a year. Even Maria goes for the quality family time.

There were these little happy moments, but things were never great at Lewisburg. At best, they were good. They were about to get worse. Much worse.

Chapter Eighteen
How Many Fish for a Hooker?

Prison is a metaphor for life,
as we cope with circumstances beyond our control
and try to live a positive and productive life,
despite an unforgiving and uncompassionate environment.

Dear Friends,

It's been several weeks since the last update. Conditions here have deteriorated and I haven't been up to writing about this place. Officials have imposed a series of actions to punish everyone for the actions of a few bad people. Here's the list:

1. Visitation has been suspended for the past month, so we haven't been able to visit face to face with family and friends. We just heard that the ban will be extended for another month, meaning that it will be at least 8 weeks that we are cut off from family. A friend's wife recently gave birth to their first child and they were scheduled to visit last month. It's a sad situation, and one that we simply can't understand.

2. The bathroom doors were removed...can you imagine that!? Sleep has been tough enough with all the snorers and noises, but now we have to deal with the bright lights from the bathroom as well as the sounds and smells from the toilets. This can't be very sanitary. The toilets are the industrial type which sound like a jet engine when flushed. People use them throughout the

nights making sleep an impossibility. I've been averaging only 4 hours a night.

3. They turned off the TVs (which I don't watch) and disconnected the ice machine, resulting in a lot of food and milk being thrown out.

4. Inmates had built a two-level mini-house for the cats to live in. There are about 15 cats here, and officials had the house crushed and removed, leaving the cats homeless. I guess they also like punishing innocent little animals.

5. As you know, we haven't had heat in months, and now that the weather has warmed up, we have heat but no air conditioning.

6. There was a major shakedown last week in the housing units as everyone was thrown out of the units while a team of cops and dogs trashed the unit looking for contraband. They totally trashed our cubicle, throwing everything from our locker on the floor as well as our clothes and papers. It took the three of us three hours to clean it up, as everything was co-mingled.

You may be asking why they would do this. Good question. Apparently last month someone from the other housing unit snuck in a woman (don't ask me how) and the guards missed finding her during their rounds. I don't know anything more other than several guys were hauled away. What I don't understand is why they would punish all the people who had nothing to do with this. Obviously they caught the ring leaders. Somehow they must think that we can use peer pressure to influence the action of other inmates. However, this is not some type of "team" environment where we can have a meeting to pull everyone together.

This is prison. The fact is there are some inmates (which I can assure you prison officials know who they are) who don't belong in a camp. The punitive actions only cause resentment and unrest with the rest of the population. All I can do is shake my head in amazement.

As you can surmise I have been struggling with the environment. I keep reminding myself that this place is much better than the Philadelphia detention center and that this is just a temporary speed-bump in my life. I will be going to home confinement at the end of July— less than 80 days. I will be working at two places: Summit Fitness and ACAC, and am excited to get back into the real world. I know this experience has changed me...just hoping it's changed me for the better.

Not much else new or exciting. As the weather has warmed I've been spending more time outside. The softball league started and we're off to a 6 & 0 start. I guess the Nationals aren't so bad after all. I'm playing first base and having a blast...even though I'm one of the oldest players. Prison softball is insane!! It has that Longest Yard feeling to it. There are two sets of bleachers which are usually filled—one always full of Latinos who heckle everyone ...all game long! Everyone heckles everyone...even within your own team. I like playing 1st base so I can trash talk the runners. My goal is not to get injured and so far so good, although my body is sore after every game. It's a long season, with 24 games before the playoffs begin.

All teachers/tutors were forced to attend a two-day training program to teach us how to be better tutors. It was a waste of taxpayers' money. It was taught by a retired grandmother (a very nice lady) who had no knowledge of what we do or how the program works. When we told her that her curriculum was not applicable to what we do she said, "Oh well, I'm here so let's go through it. I need to put 12 hours in to get paid and this will pay for my trip to Alaska this summer."

Hate to keep harping on this subject, but the amount of waste in the government is staggering. Waste is institutionalized within the system. I'm sure the BOP feels good that it "trained" its tutors and will report how they are "investing" in education.

As to the smuggled woman...

We had two dorms. One was nicknamed "the ghetto" or "the hood" and there always seemed to be something strange going on over there. That's where Bull lived. I was glad my unit was relatively sane. Eventually we heard that some of the guys in "the hood" managed to smuggle in a prostitute—and got away with it at the time. There was a gang-bang of sorts in prison! Apparently they had arranged for friends on the outside to pay her, but she was upset that she didn't get paid enough, as her clients made her work "overtime," so she contacted the warden to complain and demand her money. The warden obviously didn't take it well that some hooker wanted him to collect her pay.

At times I was able to deal with the stupidities and other times, when they piled up too much, I felt the need to rant. As aggravating as it was, I tried not to complain about it in my blogs—well not complain too much.

I started walking the track with a couple of students and am learning about life on the "streets." Boy, have we lived a sheltered life. One guy has been shot 5 times (he showed me his scars), kidnapped, and his family bound and tied up in a home invasion. The amount of money to be made is staggering, and no wonder it's hard to walk away from it to a normal job (especially without a high school diploma). They both seem committed to start a new life without the drug trade and I wish them the best of luck as they re-enter the world.

Despite the realities of prison life, there are moments of inspiration, especially when dealing with people one-on-one. There is a sense of satisfaction watching people work through their issues through yoga and meditation. At Lewisburg, most of us walk a fine line between falling into despair or embracing our circumstances, and it's nice to see people utilize these tools as they try to find their way. For me the last few weeks have blurred that line. As previously mentioned, it's sometimes difficult to "walk the walk" and practice what I preach.

Although my sad email was not a plea for sympathy and support, that is how my friends responded and I was grateful for it.

This experience has taught me that there's a fine line between a healthy attitude and depression. I am fortunate in having a relatively light sentence, yet struggle not to let the environment bring me down. Think about how hard it is for people with 3- to 10-year sentences to remain positive. There is an inmate who arrived 3 months ago for a 3-year sentence who has been a rock of stability. He's a minister who leads the Christian prayer services and bible school and who inmates often turn to when they are hurting. The minister has fallen into depression dealing with the lack of compassion and un-Christian-like behavior that I've previously highlighted. We sometimes walk the track together and I know he's hurting...he's such a good man.

Thought for the week:

Resentment or grudges do no harm to the person against whom you hold these feelings, but every day and every night of your life, they are eating at you. (Source: Norman Vincent Peale)

Softball season is in full swing. We are 8 & 1 and so far no serious injuries! This is the wild west of softball ... kind of like a cross between the Bad News Bears and Gladiator. If you can play softball in prison, you can play anywhere. There's the right fielder...a Muslim guy named Omar who has never played baseball before and has become a legend for his inability to hustle after anything. Every ball hit his way becomes a home run as he leisurely strolls to retrieve the ball. He now has a dedicated group of fans who enjoy his "inspired" level of play. I am playing well, holding down first base. However after hitting a double on a controversial play, the second baseman argued with the umpire, saying he tagged the "old guy" out. It took a while to realize that I was the "old guy." Then there's the story from last season of a transgender inmate named Marsha (previously Marvin) who didn't have time to complete the sex change surgery before going to prison (i.e. his plumbing was not yet changed). Apparently he was a heck of a player who also had nice breasts!

The saga of the homeless cats continues...A few cats had their litter so there are now a bunch of homeless kittens. An inmate was asked to remove the kittens and instead he hid them. Apparently this led to an argument with the CO so he was taken to the hole. There are 4 cats and 3 kittens left. We don't know what happened to the others. Some of the men have been taking care of them providing them milk, leftovers (although even the cats refuse to eat the tube steak).

Of all of the sad chapters of my stay at Lewisburg, one of the worst was the removal of the cats. Losing my brother was sad, but inevitable and due to no one's act of deliberate cruelty. Getting rid of the cats was some human's choice to be inhumane. Those cats (or their parents) had welcomed me to Lewisburg and given me something to smile and cry about when I very much needed it. They provided so much joy for so many of the men. It is hard to stay depressed when you are playing with a kitten. The men I saw who seemed to be the most depressed—and there were plenty here—were the ones who seemed most drawn to the cats. They spent what little money they had to get the cats some real food once in a while, and they received licks and purrs in return.

There were rumors that the cats were supposedly removed for health reasons—they might have rabies or other diseases. If that were truly the case then why just dump the cats? Why not call the local SPCA or Humane Society and have someone come get them? The cats were very tame and friendly for what were essentially semi-feral cats. I felt terrible and I know a lot of guys felt worse. It was like something out of a Steinbeck novel, where the big man refuses to be cruel to defenseless little animals and pays the price for it. It was another lost opportunity to teach a lesson in kindness to men who could use it. Instead, it reinforced that brutality was the way to go.

I was leaving soon but knew so many people would be stuck in a place that was so full of heartlessness. As happy as I was to be going home, it was sad to know that this dark world would continue. I wanted to share as many lessons as I could so that my friends and family could get the benefits of what I was learning without ever having to experience such an awful place firsthand.

Dear Friends,

Wow, mid-June already! I hope the summer is off to a great start. Mid-June means 1 1/2 months left in Lewisburg! Hard to believe that the end is in sight. The weather has been great so lots of time outdoors and a chance to find a quiet spot on the grass to get away from the mayhem...and it is mayhem. I continue to shake my head at the way this place is run (and even why it exists) and you've heard many of the stories. However with the end in sight I've gotten a second wind, as it is much easier keeping calm and patient knowing that this will soon be a part of my history. I know this has been a life-changing experience but I believe I will leave here still optimistic about human nature and the potential of the human spirit even if my faith in the government and our system of justice has been broken.

It's easy to fall down and get depressed (as you have seen me do several times). One of my bunkies, Smitty, has become depressed. He has 4 kids and is trying to adopt 4 foster kids (brothers and sisters) who have been living with his family coming out of an abusive family situation. He has the added stress of convincing "the system" that he and his wife are fit parents despite the fact he's in jail.

I was often asked to help with resumes, cover letters, and general job and life advice. I wished I had more resources with which to help these men who so desperately needed it. Many of them had never had a job and had only operated on the black market, so trying to create a resume that was not a complete pack of lies was tricky. Who could they list as references? A drug connection to whom they had been a reliable supplier?

I felt bad leaving some of these guys who were on the brink of changing their lives. I wondered if anyone else would take an interest and work as hard for them. I was hoping these men who wanted so badly to change their lives would not slide back to their old ways if no one helped them. Was it any wonder the recidivism rates are so high?

As I closed in on my release date, yet another tragedy was to befall my family. At the end of June, my mother suddenly fell ill. I tried for a furlough to go see her, but was denied due to a myriad of the excuses about paperwork. I tried to reason with them that I was being sent to house arrest at the end of July, that it was clear I was a model prisoner with a really good reputation in prison, and I was so close to getting out that there was no way I'd mess that up by not returning for those last few weeks.

I was hoping and praying that she could somehow hang on until my release, but that was not to be. It was devastating to have missed yet another important moment in my family. I felt so powerless and useless at times like this.

Chapter Nineteen
More Losses for Mr. Demeanor

Try to see yourself moving in slow motion
and you can see, experience, and savor every detail.

Dear Friends,

A heartfelt thank you for your prayers, cards, and
support in memory of my mother's passing. Even though
she was 82 years old, her passing was sudden and came
as a shock. I was unable to attend the funeral, but by
all accounts the services were beautiful and befitting
of who she was.

I've been able to maintain a positive perspective. Such
is life and yet another example of why we should enjoy
each precious moment and live in the present. As I hit
the final stretch of my time in Lewisburg, I came upon
the following which resonated with me: "Endurance is
patience concentrated," by Thomas Carlyle.

As soon as I heard that my mother had taken seriously and suddenly
ill, I asked for a furlough to go see her. It was denied. And suddenly my
mother was dead.

As happened when my brother passed, I was touched by the
outpouring of sympathy I got from the guys. Now that many of
the men knew me and liked me, I got many long hugs and people
volunteering their shoulder if I needed to cry. I was touched by their
outpouring of pure compassion and empathy.

My family was so sure I would get home for the funeral that they
pulled out my suit and had everything ready for me. Then the prison
authorities once again said no.

Some of my friends, including Bull, were surprised that I wasn't more angry or bitter at the prison authorities. I was not happy about it, but what could I do?

I couldn't control whether they let me go to her funeral. I couldn't force them to. I walked around the track, and tried to mourn as best I could. I snuck into the chapel to meditate. I had long talks with Bull about it—he had also lost his mom while he was in Lewisburg, so knew what I was going through. I could be authentic with Bull; at this point we had no pretense. I was grateful for his support, as well as that which I got from my yoga classes.

It was often difficult at times like this to not go on a rant against the administration, against the unfeeling COs. But that anger and resentment only changed *me*—not the system and not the guards. And by this time I was well aware of my position as a role model for Bull and others. I wanted to try to set a good example and be more yoga-like: accept it, control what I can, let go of things I can't. What good did it do to fight and argue? As Yogi Mike, I had to try to live up to my philosophy, and I'd remind myself that this was a chance to practice yoga.

I wrote about this to my friends:

It's easy to be philosophical the closer I get to my "Independence Day." I'm the next person in the group I hang with to be leaving. It's a weird feeling as people are generally happy for you, yet there seems to be a bit of jealousy that I will have my freedom and they won't. Freedom is something we take for granted...believe me, I won't take it for granted anymore.

Maintaining a healthy perspective is also important. While I may complain about how unfair my 9-month sentence may have been, people here can't believe how "lucky" I am to "only" have 9 months in prison. It doesn't matter what was your crime—only what is your time! The fact that I have a responsible corp. officer (with no criminal intent) misdemeanor is irrelevant to people.

Life continues to chug along relatively unchanged, although the stories continue. I continue to teach a bunch of pre-GED students off-hours. I've been swamped with inmates looking for tutoring help...most of whom are not my formal students. It's a satisfying feeling being sought out to help them, but also a sad commentary on the quality of the education program. Despite my complaints about low pay and antiquated learning tools, I've enjoyed the job and the close bond formed with my students in and out of the classroom. I've learned more from them about different cultures and life than the book knowledge they've learned from me.

The other programs are running smoothly and I'm now confident that the yoga and meditation classes will continue after I'm gone. I have 5 students ready to take over. My yoga friends can understand why I'm so passionate about these programs. I've experienced significant personal growth in dealing with my own issues. Seeing people develop positive coping mechanisms in a stressful environment is a powerful motivator to continue in this direction once I'm free.

In no particular order, here are a few amusing tidbits:

a) New mattresses (I use the term "mattress" loosely) were given to inmates in the drug program. The problem is that they are only 24" wide, while the frame is 30." A normal single mattress is 36" wide. Many inmates literally can't fit on them, let alone even think about rolling around. I could write a book about the waste and ineptitude of the prison system, but you already know this.

b) An inmate fell asleep with a cell phone in his hand, which was easy pickings for the CO, who caught him during the 2 a.m. count. He was hauled away in the middle of the night. He could probably get a gig on "World's Dumbest Criminals."

c) There was another shakedown of our housing unit where everyone had to leave the building while a team of cops searched for contraband, yet one oblivious inmate (from the drug program) went into the housing unit (which is off limits to people in the drug program) and literally walked into a cop. He was shackled and taken to the hole...another candidate for "World's Dumbest Criminals."

d) One of our card players, Papa John, has a bowel control problem and continually passes gas, especially while walking, so his name has been changed to "Drive-By John." People literally step aside when they see him coming to avoid the stink!

e) No one uses their real name. I'm known as either Yogi, Mr. Demeanor, or The Zen Master. My buddies include: Joey the Clown, Mickey Numbers, Bull, Ireland, Florida Joe, Mr. Roper, Moe Moe, Big D, Biggie, Pug, Big Money, Little Money...I could go on forever.

That's all for now. Thank you for your continued interest in my welfare. It will be so nice to communicate with you more directly.

As I got closer to my release date, I had to take the mandatory reentry classes. I thought I had endured some endless and pointless meetings in the corporate world, but these were even worse. It was almost not worth getting out of prison if this torture was the price I had to pay. The people the prison brought in were apparently not living in the same world as the men leaving prison, as the material presented was totally irrelevant to the information these men needed: how to apply for subsidized housing, food stamps, and the very basic necessities to live. Instead they were given strategies for negotiating a lease or working with a real estate agent. The instructors made passing reference to how to find an apartment, but when someone asked how one could get money for a deposit or find a place to stay until they found an apartment, the teachers could only shrug.

Some of these guys had been in so long they had never used a cell phone, let alone experienced a smartphone. I couldn't blame them for wanting to use one of the purloined phones floating around camp. There were so many practical things they would need to know to make it on the outside, and these classes offered no information along those lines.

There was a parenting course taught by someone from the outside that I heard actually was good. So many of these guys had been neglectful because they themselves had had neglectful parents. They had never learned the first thing about how to take care of kids. I had regrets about not being home enough for my daughters, but they knew I loved them and would be there for them, and I had as role models two of the best parents in the world—my own. I may not have always been able to do the right thing, but at least I knew what the right thing was.

As my release date approached, I followed camp tradition and started giving away my possessions. The books, extra toiletries, and other personal items I had accumulated weren't worth much, but to people who had almost nothing, they were valuable. I was touched by how many guys cried as I said my good-byes. I knew I had made a positive impact on some lives and hoped that some of the seeds I had planted would continue to bear fruit after I was gone.

I thought about my time in the FDC and camp and realized I had been given an amazing opportunity to learn about myself and other people in a way I never could have otherwise. I saw a side of myself that I hadn't before. I found street skills and survivor instincts I didn't know I had. I went from being a privileged white guy to being a minority in the FDC, and gained a better appreciation of what real minorities go through in their everyday lives. I thought I knew a bit about discrimination from watching how differently my daughter Maria, who is half-black, was treated than my daughter Erin, who is all Caucasian. But Maria was shielded from some of society's racism by our upper-middle-class family. So many of the guys I met at the FDC and at Lewisburg had clearly ended up where they were for no good reason other than being black or Latino; any similar white defendant would have gotten a slap on a wrist.

And although I might complain that I had been singled out for a jail sentence that no one else got for my level of misdemeanor, I could be sure it was not because of the color of my skin. I had no doubt I was afforded better treatment by the COs in Lewisburg, and I knew I had a secure life, well out of harm's way, with money, a home, and family and friends, to which I would return. The same could not be said for too many of my fellow inmates.

Some of the guys I worked with were just starting on their journey, whether to literacy or spirituality, and I hoped they would continue. I felt bad I was leaving them when there was so much more work to be done. But I was done with this part of my own journey and had to go.

Dear Friends,

I thought this day would never come! It's Thursday, July 19, so only 5 more days until I'm out of here. On Monday morning I will lose access to email and the phone so wanted to share these thoughts while I can. Surprisingly, these past few weeks have passed quickly.

I wanted to thank each of you for your unwavering support through the highs and lows and everything in between. Your letters, cards, books, and more importantly your emotional support made a huge difference. You were my connection to the outside world and a source of stability and a calming influence. It's somewhat ironic that it took going away to prison to get closer to many of you. I was taken aback by your concern, prayers, and condolences for my mom. It was extraordinarily painful not attending the funeral, especially after losing my brother Bob. Yet I felt a genuine warmth and sense of peace knowing the loving support she had. You all provided a "virtual" community for me while dealing with the day-to-day trials and tribulations in an environment desperately lacking compassion. Thank you from the bottom of my heart.

I plan to reach out to you once I get settled back home and happily will be able to contact you directly!

Many thoughts and lessons learned run through my mind and in no particular order:

We don't need material things to be happy. I came to this prison with literally nothing, and 8 months later leave with a small box of personal effects: legal papers, 3 books, a plastic coffee cup and a pair of sweat pants. Yet I don't feel deprived. In many ways I feel blessed having been able to become an avid reader and having the opportunity to better know myself.

Family and friends are precious. Sounds obvious but I think we sometimes take them for granted. Maybe it takes being removed from them or losing them to fully appreciate how they shape and affect our lives. My situation may be extreme but it's a case study in the positive influence of family bonds.

There is a fine line between depression and joy. The human spirit is strong, but it can be broken if not nurtured. There are people here with 10-year sentences who are full of life and carry an upbeat vibe with them, while others with much shorter sentences seem to carry a heavy burden on their shoulders.

So many people are bitter about so many things...this is not healthy. While I have complained about many unjust things about Lewisburg, I do not leave a bitter person. Rather than bitter, I hope I leave here a "better" person.

Yoga—the power is tangible, real, positive, and universal. Lewisburg has afforded the opportunity for a deep dive into the 8 Limbs of Yoga to see firsthand the power it has to improve lives and to have people become comfortable in their own skin. I've seen people of diverse ethnic, religious and economic backgrounds address their inner demons (be they guilt, shame, depression, unworthiness, etc.) in a direct and positive manner. This process of self-reflection can lead to life-changing transformation.

We adapt to our environment. At the end of the day, people are people. We all come from different life circumstances and have made decisions that have affected the quality of our lives. Some of us were given life opportunities while others are less fortunate. Yet I believe there is a core life force or a soul that connects us. I've been fortunate to see both sides of the spectrum from living as a corporate CEO to being an inmate teaching semi-literate inmates. One group is certainly not better than the other... in fact, many of my students regret some of their life decisions and seem to be on a path toward a healthy and rewarding life. I have enjoyed being with this group more than at the executive dinners.

Cultural differences are huge but overcome-able (is this a word!?). It took a while to adjust to the living conditions where a sink has multiple uses...to wash your face, wash clothes, wash dishes, dispose of food, and cook food (run hot water over food wrapped in plastic). Poor hygiene habits are a turnoff, but do not define the person. I've formed bonds with people from the opposite spectrum of society and as a result, hopefully, have more understanding of others.

Everyone makes mistakes. We just don't pay for our mistakes in the same way. Many people here are truly remorseful for their crimes and have paid a debt far greater than prison time: loss of family, financial ruin, loss of self-worth. I walk away less judgmental about the actions of others and more aware of how my actions impact others.

My time in Lewisburg makes me more appreciative of the sacrifices our military families make in serving our country, with soldiers put in harm's way for extended periods of time away from their families.

I still believe in the spirit and greatness of this country, but have been profoundly disappointed in the waste, corruption, and loss of human potential in how the prison system operates. The injustice of the justice system combined with the lack of any sense of compassion goes against the core values of how the country was founded. Quite frankly, this system is hopelessly broken and needs new leadership, ideas, and energy to reduce the amount of corruption and to help rehabilitate inmates while they are being punished. I would hope that someday the prison system could be part of the solution instead of the problem.

Last night during yoga class, a tremendous thunderstorm blew in, knocking out power. We continued our practice as flashes of lightning lit up the gym then quickly returned us to dark shadows. Bodies appeared as moving through a strobe light. Loud thunder blasts echoed through the gym, providing a dramatic effect to our airplane and half-moon poses, resulting in a deeply spiritual and emotional experience. After class the eight of us looked at each other knowing that we had just experienced something special. I think this may have been a metaphor for my time here. I leave you with a quote from T.S. Eliot: "What we call the beginning is often the end. And to make an end is to make a beginning. The end is where we start from." I look forward to seeing and talking to you on the "other" side.

Love & gratitude.
Mike

Chapter Twenty
Free Hugs

With the right attitude and perspective,
adversity evolves into wisdom.
All of life's events make us who we are,
and we are not defined by any one thought or action.

My daughters picked me up around 10 a.m. and brought a change of clothes, short pants, a pullover knit shirt, sneakers, and my favorite baseball cap. They felt so good, although they were baggy after all of my weight loss. Maria was wearing a T-shirt that said "Free Hugs." As if the sentiment of freedom couldn't make me any happier, it brought a huge smile to my face. My head was spinning with so many emotions that tears ran down my cheeks. The COs who processed me out gave me friendly words of advice: "Don't come back! We don't want to see you again!"

I'll never forget the surreal feeling of walking out the front door and into my car. And just like that I drove past the Big House, down the hill, and back into the real world.

The first thing we did was drive two minutes to the nearby Dunkin' Donuts. It was crazy, but of all the creature comforts I had been denied for the last nine months, what I missed most was good coffee. I never thought I would taste anything so wonderful again.

Then we set off to drive to Philadelphia. Although I would still be under the supervision and control of the Federal court for another three months, it felt amazing to be off the small compound that had been my home for so long.

Like when I arrived at Lewisburg, I had not realized the amount of tension I was holding in parts of my body until I began to unwind. The beautiful, rolling hills of central Pennsylvania are so much more enjoyable from the window of my family's car than from the windows of a prison bus with an unknown destination.

Erin and Maria had brought me a duffle bag packed with a few days' worth of my clothes and some toiletries for what I hoped would be just a short stay at the halfway house. The house was in a bad part of north Philadelphia, but with all of its restrictions it would still seem like paradise compared to my last accommodations. And if all went well, I might be there only for a weekend and then would be released to house arrest in my own home. We made good time and got lucky: the man who had to process me was still there and said he'd do my paperwork right away.

The girls had planned to drive home and come back for me whatever day I was let go. He let me call my daughters and tell them not to go too far—I'd be released within several hours. I was almost more worried about my girls in this part of town than my getting stuck overnight in the halfway house. After I did a drug and alcohol test and some paperwork, my daughters picked me up and we went home.

It felt so odd to get home. It felt so good to walk in the door, but I somehow expected something more. I wanted to hear violins or have a rainbow appear above the house.

I wanted to kiss my bed and then I wanted to sleep. A lot. So many things felt wonderful, especially sleeping in a nice bed on soft sheets. I had spent so many hours dreaming of being home and not worrying and feeling safe—and now here I was!

When I awoke the next morning, I had a brief, mild panic because I couldn't find my shower slippers. Then I remembered I didn't need them: no scum lurked in my bathroom.

I would have many limitations on my life for a while, but compared to where I had been, they seemed petty and annoying, but not cumbersome. I had to call to let my supervising officer know when I left for work. I had to call and let him know when I arrived at work. If I wanted to go anywhere besides the straight shot from home to work or back again—the grocery store, a doctor's appointment—I had to get advance permission.

They had the authority to show up at my house or work at any time and make sure I was where I was supposed to be. They could order me to take a drug or alcohol test at any time. This I found interesting. My crime was not drug or alcohol related, so why would they suddenly think I would start abusing either? I did get a couple of calls to report within two hours for a urine test, and one night they did ring my doorbell at 2 a.m. to make sure I was home. I was glad for small favors: the cars and people they sent to my home or work to check up on me were unmarked—no uniforms or police cars. My boss at work knew my situation, but the parole officers supervising me never revealed to the people at the front desk or anyone else who they were or why they wanted to see me.

— — —

I thought I would come out of Lewisburg and just be walking on air—all the weight would be lifted and I would be literally and figuratively home free. But after a few days of feeling wonderful at being out, things starting sinking. I had a much harder time readjusting than I ever thought I would. I didn't know why. It wasn't survivor's guilt, although little things could send my thoughts flying back to my friends at Lewisburg. I'd see food in the grocery store and think, "Bull would love this!" I'd have Mexican food and wonder if the guys were making burritos on an iron. In some odd way I missed it.

My friends and family on the outside were all eager to see me and wanted to have a big party to welcome me back to the real world, but I said no. I wasn't ready to face a lot of people, and I quietly told a few who were sort of insisting: this is not a celebration—I am just trying to get on with my life. It was strange; I could go to work and see a good many people in the gym and in my yoga classes, but they didn't interact with me on a personal level. I wasn't ready to really talk to people yet.

I found myself having a mild paranoia: the stigma of going to the grocery store and being recognized from TV or the many newspaper articles. It was ridiculous given how long it had been and how unimportant the story was to most people. It wasn't as though I was Bernie Madoff or Jeffrey Dahmer; unlike them, my photo had not repeatedly been in every magazine and on every newscast for months.

I wondered if the students in my yoga class knew where I had been or talked to each other about me and my criminal past. If anyone asked where I'd been, I answered, "I was away," in a vague manner that left little room for follow-up questions. Synthes is near the yoga studio where I was teaching, and I had people in my classes who used to work for me coming to my yoga class—they did know where I'd been. They were sympathetic and compassionate, wishing me well in an awkward sort of way, not knowing exactly what to say or how to say it. Some said it was good to have me back, and I would answer, "It's great to be back," without going into any detail.

— — —

I found the yoga classes I was teaching to be the same and yet completely different from the ones I had taught before I had been in prison. After practicing yoga without a mat, yoga clothes or a lemon in my water bottle, I got something totally different out of the poses than I used to, and now felt that passion and fire deep within me even as I taught suburban housewives. It was so much more real and meaningful now, even if I wasn't always successful in sharing that deep emotion with my students, who were rushing back to their lives.

Outside of work and yoga, I was struggling. Life in prison is very simple: I couldn't control anything in prison, so I just had to cope with whatever came my way. Now I had to start making my own decisions. All of the stuff I left behind was still there—in fact, it was worse because of neglect. My marriage, my relationship with my daughters, what to do about a job…A thousand personal things needed attention.

I found myself nagged by another thought—the worse I felt about my situation, the worse I felt about myself. I was Yogi Mike. I had my act together. I was the guy everyone turned to for comfort. I was the rock in the troubled stream of Lewisburg—but now I was out and I didn't know what to do with myself. I felt bad that I couldn't do for myself what I had done for so many at the camp. A basic tenet of yoga is self-acceptance and self-love. The frustrating part of this was I knew what was going on, but I couldn't find the strength or fortitude to do something about it.

In my troubled state, I couldn't even tell anyone what was wrong. I wanted to be the strong one and didn't want to admit that part of me was afraid to face the world, unsure of my next steps. I was the one who guided others on the path and now couldn't find it for myself. I felt guilty that I wasn't instantly euphorically happy and eager to embrace the real world and my family and friends who had been so loyal and supportive while I was inside.

During this period I would wake up at 5:30 a.m., seemingly keeping the same schedule as at Lewisburg. I'd have a cup of coffee and sit on my deck enjoying the solitude and nature. This was a time of self-assessment, with a wide range of emotions spanning from fear and uncertainty to joy. I half expected some variety of epiphany to come to me, but it didn't. I watched small animals play in the yard and wondered what to do with myself. During my time at Lewisburg, I truly felt that I'd *found* myself and was so convinced that I would live an authentic life and be true to who I thought I was. Why was I now doubting all of this?

In retrospect, perhaps I should have gone on blogging as I had while I was in Lewisburg. While I was locked up, it felt good to vent and release my thoughts on paper—or, well, at least pixels. Now that I could pick up a phone and call the people to whom I'd been writing, now that I could invite them over and see them face-to-face, it seemed odd to go on writing. Besides, what did I really have to complain about—I was home, I had my freedom, I could buy and eat any food I wanted, I could sleep in a comfortable bed. It seemed selfish to ask them to listen to me whine now that everything was good—or should have been good. I understood their putting up with my venting while I was in prison, but now it would seem petulant and childish.

For the first month or so that I was home, I saw only Colleen and another longtime friend and a few family members. I was saying no to many visitors.

My father came to stay with me for a few days. While my house arrest continued, I couldn't go visit him and we wanted to reconnect. It was a bittersweet visit. I was shocked by how much he had aged mentally and physically.

We had heartfelt discussions about how our lives had changed: what life after Lewisburg would be like for me and what life without my mother was for him. He was definitely feeling down and not the same guy I had left behind. I wished I was in a better place myself to be stronger and in a position to help him. But while sinking in quicksand, it is hard to save anyone else.

My parents had been married for over sixty years. In addition to missing the emotional side of their marriage, he missed the practical side as well. They had a very traditional post-World War II marriage, and he was struggling with things like doing laundry, shopping, and cooking—things that he took for granted because my mother had always handled them so well. I had to give him housekeeping tips for bachelors.

I was glad to hear that he was still doing yoga three or four times a week at his retirement community. I had gotten both of my parents to try it during my purgatory years. Mom loved her tai chi classes and Dad was now deep into yoga. Obviously, a very gentle sort of yoga given his age and that of the other residents of that senior community, but he truly enjoyed the controlled breathing, stretching, movement, and mindfulness. He said yoga was helping him come to terms with my mom's passing as well as helping keep his mind from deteriorating.

While my father was visiting me, I felt I had to be somewhat upbeat for his sake. After he left, I was even more down and feeling lost. I didn't even know how to explain to anyone what I was going through. It wasn't like a veteran returning from Iraq, in which case people might have some concept of what I had been through and why I might not want to open up about it. And I hadn't done anything patriotic or heroic; I had been to prison.

It has been said that we are all faking it—adults, parents, husbands, wives, and CEOs who pretend to know it all, don't. They are just better at bluffing. But now minus the titles and trappings, who was I? I was no longer a husband or CEO. I had no standing in the community. With my mask ripped away, I was having a harder time faking it.

— — —

While I was trying not to drown in Lewisburg, I could delay making any major decisions. Now I was treading water, expending a lot of energy and not getting anywhere.

Jenny was hopeful that once I got out and put the worst behind me, things would be different. She had remained supportive throughout my sentencing and incarceration, but I had told her that we were not going to get back together, and now I had to deal with the mess of getting divorced. I knew I had hurt Jenny and didn't want this to be more painful than it was already going to be for her, for our daughters, for the rest of our families, and for me. It was hard enough to register a car while I was in prison; I couldn't imagine handling the complications of a divorce, but now the time to face the unpleasantness was here. In Lewisburg, I could find things to occupy me—whether it was tutoring or playing softball—it kept me from really facing my problems and my future. Now I had to.

One thing that the clean break of the prison had given me was clarity. All the yoga I did in prison helped give me the strength to confront the fact that I was no longer in love. I am a pleaser, so for years had pretended to be happy, but it had been years since I last had really been happy. It had nothing to do with my legal problems, or losing my job. This malaise had been brewing for years before any of that. I still wanted to please Jenny, my girls, and the rest of my family, so it was stressful knowing that this was going to hurt a lot of people, and between my incarceration and the loss of my brother and mother, my family had already been through a lot in the last year.

With a strict Catholic upbringing, divorce had never seemed like an option. No one in my family had ever gotten a divorce. Yoga and meditation and all of the personal growth I had experienced had given me the strength to be able to tell Jenny that I wanted a divorce, and now I had to finish it. There is the line from the old song—you can't please everyone, so you've got to please yourself. I knew I would not be any good to anyone else, least of all myself, if I didn't take care of this.

Toward the end I was not committed to doing a good job in my marriage. I was acting as a good husband and good father, and I tried to be all of those things, although I traveled too much to have done as good a job as I could have, as I should have, as I wished I had. Being away on business trips so much, it was easier to fake it when I got home, but being around so much during the purgatory years had made it impossible to pretend any longer. In reality, I came to understand that I really wasn't a good husband to Jenny. That's the cold, hard fact that I had to digest, embrace, and eventually let go of.

— — —

Along with dealing with the divorce, I had to figure out what to do next. Before I even started job hunting, through personal connections I got offers to return to the corporate world. Had that path been an easy, open highway, I might have actually done it. What else was I supposed to do? What else did I know how to do?

While I was still in Lewisburg, I had been contacted by a former board member from Synthes. He asked if I might be interested in going to work for his company. When I got out, I talked to him again and tried to arrange a flight to Florida for the final interview and expected job offer.

The parole department encouraged—almost demanded—that I work during this period. They were happy that I had a job as a yoga instructor and personal trainer. However, they balked when I requested permission to fly to Florida for this interview. The parole officer complained about the amount of paperwork involved to get approval for travel outside of the court's regional jurisdiction and denied my request.

Wasn't the idea for me to reenter society as a productive member? But they would rather have me making barely better than minimum wage (and paying commensurately low taxes) than having me jump back into the corporate world at a decent pay grade. There was the other barrier to reentering the corporate world: due to my conviction, I was forbidden from working in any health care-related industry for five years.

I had lots of experience in the medical industry, and lots of contacts who would have made getting a job there easy. While these roadblocks were starting to frustrate me, it suddenly hit me. Maybe I wasn't meant to go down that road! I think at times the universe, or god, or fate or _____ (fill in the blank) is trying to tell us things. And if you don't listen the first time, it says it louder the next time. Now the universe was pretty much yelling in my ear: DON'T GO BACK TO THE CORPORATE WORLD!

Some people may not buy the notion that "the universe" is trying to tell me something or "god is sending me a message," but even stripped of any metaphysics, there comes a time when you start noticing things you hadn't noticed before. Perhaps you're thinking of buying a new Acura RL and now everywhere it seems you're seeing them. An Acura parks next to you at the gym. An Acura merges in front of you on the highway. Were there always that many Acuras around? Probably. But now that they've entered your consciousness as you consider your purchase, you see them in a way you hadn't before. Even in the color you like.

It's hard to know whether the universe is sending you a message, or if some part of your brain is finally focusing on messages that have always been there. Does it even matter, as long as you recognize that input and act on it when it arrives?

One day after yoga, it suddenly hit me like a two-by-four upside the head, and I was finally ready to listen to this message. Once I accepted the message, there came another more pressing question: If I didn't go back into the corporate world, what was I supposed to do? I wanted to find space to think.

Chapter Twenty-One
Transformation

Transcend your judgments.
Judgments come from the head;
freedom and love come from the heart.

After my month of house arrest was over and I could travel freely, I started going to my regular yoga class in West Chester with Colleen. The classes helped me start to feel a little more human and ease back into society and socializing. I felt so different about so many things now. For years I had been sort of a closet yoga guy, but after a decade of upheavals, I now proudly carried my mat and my status as a yogi.

I wanted yoga to give me the answers, but sometimes fate takes a hand in other ways. I had a strong desire to get away from it all and just, literally, sail away. It was one of the many things I longed for when I was incarcerated. I wanted to be on the open sea, working as crew on a traditional sailing boat. The destination wasn't as important as the journey, but the season was rapidly changing, and I knew it would soon be too cold to sail around New Jersey, so I decided to sail somewhere in the Caribbean. I Googled "sailing singles"—not looking for a date, but to find a boat that was looking for a crew member. What came up was a dating site for active singles. On a whim, being somewhat curious, I created a profile. I really didn't want to date yet; I was fresh out of prison and not yet divorced. But I was curious, so I went ahead and registered.

A surprising number of women contacted me almost immediately, but all were far away and I wasn't even sure I wanted to be in a relationship, let alone a long-distance one. A few days after joining the site, I got a message from a woman in Delaware, less than forty minutes south of me. She said she was new to the site also.

I knew nothing about online dating or its customs and protocols. The last time I had dated anyone there was no internet. I was embarrassed to admit to anyone, most of all my children, that I was exploring this world. I was going to have to blunder along on my own.

The woman's name was Beverly, and in our brief exchange of messages, we hit it off instantly. We seemed to have a lot in common, with an interest in business, an interest in spirituality, and a desire to improve ourselves.

We were both eager to talk on the phone. Of course this would involve telling her my name. She seemed like an intelligent woman and before she would agree to meet, I was sure she would Google me. I didn't know much about this new dating world, but I knew anyone with any sense would take that precaution. When we spoke on the phone, I knew before the conversation went too far I would have to unchain the elephant in the room. If I was going to date I wanted to do it with no secrets, no pretenses, no regrets.

I wasn't ready to date anyway; if the truth scared her away, so be it. I told her I was fresh out of prison, and why I had been there. She got quiet, and stayed quiet for quite a while after I told her. I didn't have more to add to my story at that point, but I couldn't take the silence any longer and said, "I completely understand if you don't want anything to do with me."

There was still silence. All I could say was, "I understand if you want to think about this." She said she did and the call ended on that awkward note. She sent me a text later that said, "There is a lot of really bad stuff out there about you." I couldn't dispute that. I had tried to avoid reading all of the bad news about me, but I knew from others that there was plenty.

She said she'd like to know more and hear my side of the story. Beverly wanted to see me in person and said she would reserve judgment until she got to know me a bit. We agreed to meet the next day in Kennett Square, a cute little town in southeastern Pennsylvania. I let her lead the conversation, and she didn't ask much about what she had read online. She was willing to see me again, so I invited her to go on a group hike the next day. I told her there would be about twenty-five people there, in case she was afraid to be alone in the woods with a stranger.

She agreed to go. It was a beautiful day, with the crisp air and bright fall colors for which Pennsylvania is rightfully famous. While staying in sight of the group, we broke off a ways from the pack so we could talk more privately. She had done a great deal of research online and was full of questions. I did my best to answer them.

"I understand if you did these things because you were lured by the money," she said.

"I'd be happy to tell you that, but I can only tell you the truth," I replied. "I didn't do the things described in the press—it's just not who I am."

Maybe this whole ugly mess would have made sense if Synthes or I or anyone had made millions, but the fact was that I was not compensated at all for the product in question and had never marketed it illegally for profit.

Beverly—this all-but-stranger—believed that I was not the evil person the articles said I was.

I also was up-front about the fact that although I had been separated for well over a year and was in the process of divorcing, I was technically still married. She seemed okay with that as well, because she planned to take things slowly.

Although we said we'd take things slowly, we actually started seeing a good deal of each other, and within two weeks, Beverly and I were planning to take a vacation together months down the road.

As we started to meet each other's friends and families, she asked me not to say anything about my past. She wanted them to get to know me before they let the prejudice that accompanies "ex-con" cloud their opinion.

Many dates later, Beverly told me that when she hung up the phone after our first call she said to herself, "That is the man I am going to marry." She also later said that I was a cheap date—she only had to pay for one month's membership to the dating site. Like me, she had fallen for the first and only person she had met from the site.

I wondered how I was so lucky to find a woman like this. She explained that she had been single for so long because she had been so busy building her own business, and hadn't found time for a husband. Beverly told friends, "I gave birth to a company instead of a child."

She wanted a man who was experienced in life as well as someone on the path to a better life as she was.

— — —

For a while, Beverly was tolerant of some of my post-prison quirks. For instance, I had developed a quasi-obsession with TV programs about prison. Shows including *Locked Up* were a form of entertainment that never would have interested me a year earlier. She was willing to listen when my thoughts drifted back to the FDC or Lewisburg. Like soldiers who had been to war, the experience was so stark and sharp that it seemed to permeate my thoughts at the oddest times. That year was such an upheaval, like a volcano that rose out of my life, that it seemed to dwarf the flat landscape that occurred before and after.

I'd look at the clock and think it was time for a stand-up count. It would get near time for our Friday night card game and I'd wonder what the guys were doing, what the iron-cooked meal du jour was. I'd look at the calendar and remember that one of my friends was getting out about now. I wondered if they would get their lives back on track. After one too many references to these things, Beverly said, "I wish you would just move on. You talk about it all the time."

It was never an intentional thought. I would just see someone being pulled over by the police and wonder what was happening—if they were about to get arrested. I would see something on TV that would spark a memory. I had to agree with Beverly, it wasn't healthy to visit those thoughts too often. In *Orange is the New Black*, Piper Kerman also wrote that it was almost impossible to go an entire day without her mind drifting back to prison. Both Piper's and my sentences were relatively short—each about a year—I couldn't imagine what a long stint would do to your mind and how much stronger that dark gravity must be to pull one back to that unhappy time and place.

Amazingly, Beverly also seemed okay with my current existential crisis. I told her I had no real job, legal matters hanging over my head from the divorce and the Synthes mess, and was still on probation. Instead of being put off by these things, she offered to help me sort out my life. She suggested I see a life coach she knew. After just a few visits with the coach, what I should be doing began to gel. The pieces had been there for a while; I just had to arrange them.

— — —

Beverly is self-motivated and spiritual in a straightforward sort of way. I tended to overanalyze things, and she was more decisive and action-oriented. Yet our overall philosophies about life were similar, and we agreed that there is more than one approach that works. She had tried traditional yoga and found it wasn't really for her, but instead became an avid practitioner of aerial yoga, the kind that looks a bit like Cirque Du Soleil.

Her approach helped me not to repeat the mistakes from my marriage. Instead of hoarding ammunition for months that built into guerilla wars, Beverly and I would sometimes argue, but we dealt with the issue quickly and directly so it didn't have time to fester into something bigger. As a result, we didn't stay mad long. We communicated in ways I never could before. Beverly and I joked that if we knew each other five years ago, we'd have killed each other; we were both such uptight, Type-A personalities.

I began to deal with a lot of my pent-up baggage of my brother, mother, and father. I was so busy dealing with more immediate problems that I never took time to grieve. Now I took that time.

I had never examined where my life went wrong in terms of my marriage or career. With the help of Beverly and the coach, I looked at those things. I realized that part of my difficulty in mentally leaving prison was that as long as I was in prison—physically or psychologically—I had a good excuse not to address my other emotional issues. Now I couldn't hide behind that shield any longer. Once I faced those issues from my past, I was ready to turn around and face my future.

— — —

I think I knew all along what I should be doing, but I just needed to hear it confirmed by someone else. The coach never told me what to do; he just helped me find the answer.

While I was still in Lewisburg, I had the idea of setting up a consulting business to help guide business executives. I had done a business plan for a company that would focus on business executives who were stressed and burnt out, and provide help with their emotional growth, family/work balance, and developing practical mindfulness for the corporate world.

I had started teaching a class at a junior college in Coatesville, a depressed area where students, like those in Lewisburg, were struggling to do something better with their lives.

When I thought back to the yoga nidra classes I taught in Lewisburg, it hit me that this was a great idea, but it was for the wrong audience. One day during yoga, I had an epiphany about working with people at risk instead of business executives: I needed to focus on people who needed it more, but couldn't afford yoga and mindfulness classes.

I had this notion while I was in Lewisburg, but until now I hadn't fully shifted gears from wanting a for-profit for execs to a nonprofit to help those who really needed it. I had been on the board of the local YMCA and another charity called Open Hearth, and knew some of the challenges inherent in running a nonprofit and having to raise money through donations and grants.

Many well-intentioned do-gooders start nonprofits, but lack business sense, something I had in abundance. I had seen many wonderful people who were committed to saving the world start charities, but had them fail because they didn't understand that to remain viable as a nonprofit, you still had to have income. Nonprofit didn't mean no money.

I had half-baked thoughts of what would become the Transformation Yoga Project (TYP), but it hadn't gelled. TYP is exactly what I thought I should be doing back then, but if anyone had asked me the details then, those pieces would not have looked like TYP. In a way, it's completely different and yet exactly what it should be. For the first time in years, I knew I was headed in the right direction and that things were going to be okay.

Ultimately it was seeing and experiencing the role that unresolved trauma plays in preventing us to become our true self, which formed the core concept of TYP. Whether in prison, juvenile detention, work or personal relationships, unresolved trauma can prevent us from experiencing the present moment in a truly nonjudgmental way. TYP was founded to address the impact trauma has on preventing us from living a full life regardless of the challenges. This eureka moment wouldn't have come without the journey through prison.

I realized that another amazing thing did come of all of this: I found myself.

My former coworker and still good friend, Jim O'Neill, said he could see I was taking baby steps toward becoming a true yogi, but if prison had not intervened and ripped me off the road I had been on, at the pace I was moving I would have died of old age before I reached the destination to which my year in hell had brought me. I was doing what I was meant to do. Jim could see it. I could see it. I was finally on the path.

Chapter Twenty-Two
Finding Myself

Listen to the universe.
It is the voice that will lead you to live your authentic life.
It sends us signals all the time.
Sometimes it takes a punch in the gut to listen to the answer you need.
You don't have to wait for the punch to live an authentic life.

It was yoga that had kept me afloat and kept me sane during my two-and-a-half-year purgatory and months of incarceration. I realized I had a chance to pay it forward and throw that life preserver to others who were struggling.

Once I decided what to do, the first person I contacted was James Fox, of the Prison Yoga Project. He had been taking yoga into California prisons, including San Quentin, for over a decade. When I heard back from him, he told me he was just about to conduct a training for volunteers working in prisons in New York City and invited me to attend.

So much of what I had figured out on my own and through trial and error at the FDC and at Lewisburg, James had known for years from his work in San Quentin, other San Francisco-area prisons, juvenile facilities, and the like. He was willing to share all that he had learned. Much of what he knew was also from experience. Now I had my own experiences to inform my teaching.

I knew from the amount of tension I stored in prison that keeping things bottled up in your tissues isn't healthy. Getting people to stop thinking so much is a big piece of what we do, whether in yoga for recovery or veterans or inmates. This problem is really acute with the veterans: they are trained to take orders and go places that common sense says you shouldn't. When they get out, they can't disconnect from suppressing the feelings of fighting their own best instincts in order to complete the mission.

Fortunately, from a scientific perspective, we are learning a great deal about how trauma impacts the mind and body. Bessel van der

Kolk, MD, has extensively studied the impact of trauma ⌐ and published a fantastic book about the mind/body connection, *Body Keeps the Score: Brain, Mind, and Body in the Healing of Trauma.* He wrote about the research showing that traumatic stress symptoms have a physiological basis. Our body has a natural survival mechanism. When under threat, it switches into "fight or flight" mode. Activation of this response comes from the sympathetic nervous system, which instinctively does what it needs to protect itself. The release of adrenaline increases the heart rate, blood pressure, and breathing as it prepares the body for action. This gives us the ability to respond to a threat without worrying much about emotion. It's a natural and healthy response to stress.

Once the body believes it is now "safe," we return to our natural state and the sympathetic nervous system becomes dormant, while the parasympathetic system returns. The parasympathetic system stimulates different physical responses and allows us to become more rational, emotional, and empathetic. Post-traumatic stress can occur when, during the fight or flight response, the person is not able to do either. The body and emotions have gone so far into the "danger" range, or stayed there for so long that it's no longer able to shift gears as it should.

The body can't naturally return to "safe" mode. Imagine you were being kidnapped and were unable to fight or otherwise escape. The adrenaline and other physical changes kick in, but ultimately there isn't a natural release, and the tension and stress become stored in the body. The result is that people with post-traumatic stress disorder (PTSD) don't feel safe, not in the community nor in their own bodies. This is why we believe that reconnecting the mind and body is so important so that there can be a proper equilibrium between the sympathetic and parasympathetic systems. Essentially, we would like our students to feel safe within their own bodies, able to make the distinction between the horrific experiences of the past and the non-threatening present moment.

There are many forms of yoga, but what seemed to work best for people dealing with stress is trauma-informed yoga practice. This type of yoga teaches us to check in and ask, "How are you feeling? Does this feel right? Do you need to back off the pose?" It is an invitation to make a conscious connection between sensations in the body and a compassionate response from the mind. The poses are designed to force the mind to focus on breathing, and the physical pose prevents the mind from wandering onto thoughts of the past or future which they don't control. Even though a student may be straining to hold a pose, focusing on the discomfort in their shoulders forces them to become aware of the body sensation and make a decision about whether they should hold the pose or back off. This keeps them in the present moment and may eventually reconnect the mind and body, ultimately allowing them to understand that they can release their thoughts and recognize that current thoughts are not the same as the original trauma they experienced.

While I laid plans for TYP, I sought out the local VA Hospital to volunteer. I couldn't wait to get involved. After navigating the somewhat frustrating clearance process, I started four classes. Veterans have a camaraderie that is special. They had served our country and many had paid a high price. These men and women were always pleasant and friendly despite dealing with heavy-duty issues. It was such a sobering experience to see firsthand the cost of war on the lives of these amazing people. Some of the veterans would want to tell me what they did in combat and the shame and regret they felt. For many, they had taken the war home with them.

Trauma is at the root of many problems leading to prison or drugs. The traumas that vets experience may have very different roots, but the negative impact on their bodies often manifests the same. People in recovery often get a glimpse of their lives through yoga; tears and small breakdowns are not uncommon.

I knew very little about addiction problems until I went to prison, where I saw so many people struggling to rid themselves of the addiction and the underlying problems that caused them to turn to drugs or alcohol. Now much of what TYP does is work with people who are trying to find a better path.

Whether in prison or a veterans' facility or recovery center, the classes themselves provide a sense of community. In places where people often feel alone and isolated, there is a "brotherhood of the mat" that helps the participants feel connected to someone or something beyond themselves. For so many whose addictions or incarceration have left them estranged from their families, it helps so much to give them a sense of belonging—if only for an hour or two a week.

Many people make the mistake of living in the past—dwelling on mistakes or things they wish they had done differently. It is also common for people at troubled places in their lives to live in the future instead of in the present. So many guys I met at Lewisburg spoke wishfully of what would happen when they were released, but I met very few who were taking any steps to create that future. I could relate because when I got out, I froze with the fear of what I should do next. Now that I had found my mission, I knew I was especially well-equipped to help others.

I had seen it in prison and I would see it often in the VA—the downside of stereotypical male role behavior—never show fear, never back down. This was true when dealing with inner-city violence and the military. I just hoped to open their eyes to the choice to do something different.

I felt energized and ready to move forward with the Transformation Yoga Project. But first I had to confront other challenges.

My father had one of the first artificial valve surgeries back in the 1960s. The artificial valve was not supposed to last for decades, so in a way he'd been on borrowed time. He got an infection from a dental treatment which led to more problems; then he collapsed.

When I got the word, we were under hurricane watch for superstorm Sandy, which was headed smack into the Jersey shore and directly toward the hospital where Dad was being treated. Since its predicted landfall was still twenty-four hours away, I drove the two hours to the hospital. The next day, my father took a turn for the worse.

When it seemed that my father was going to hang in there a while longer, Larry and I went back to our father's house to spend the night. It was strange and macabre to be sitting around in near darkness with only the faint glow of a few candles for light, and we talked about our father and his impending death. The next day we returned to the hospital through flooded and debris-strewn streets to wait by our father's bedside. He hung on for two more days, and then quietly passed away.

I had now lost three family members in less than a year, so I was very grateful that I had gotten out in time to get reacquainted with him on a new level. His was the only one of the recent family funerals at which I could share grief with my family. Part of my yoga and spiritual practice was to have no regrets and not dwell on things I couldn't change. I would miss him, of course. I tried to console myself that he had lived a loving and compassionate life, but recently he had not been happy living alone without my mom.

— — —

About this time, a challenge of a completely different nature presented itself. I accepted an invitation to speak to the Greater Philadelphia Senior Executive Group, where a friend was vice chair of their CEO Roundtable. He wanted me to tell my story. I wasn't sure I was ready to share my truth in public. I still had a hard time telling anyone I had been to prison. He convinced me that not only might it be cathartic for me but it might also help some of the other execs avoid falling into the same tiger pits I had. Fortunately, Beverly attended and provided much needed emotional support. I teared up a few times, but the overwhelming response from these CEOs was worth it. Many of them also welled up with emotion. It was all part of my journey, and convinced me I had a story to share.

Men and women who I barely knew reached out with hugs and offered their support. They understood the pressures and multitude of responsibilities facing executives and could picture themselves in the same situation.

They showed great empathy as they asked questions about the impact of the ordeal professionally and personally and many asked, "How can you not be bitter and angry?"

Some focused on the business aspect saying, "I'm going to change how I manage," or "I'm going to do a complete review of our internal controls—both the procedures and the engagement by the organization."

Others focused on the personal, saying, "I need to get my personal priorities and life in order!"

Still others sympathized that they understood how the legal process can sometimes be disconnected from discovering the truth.

And they asked many questions about what it's like to be in prison. They were curious about the logistics, food, interaction of white-collar criminals with the general population, and more. Some seemed to feel they themselves had dodged a bullet and wanted to learn without having to go through what I had. There was a lot of, "But for the grace of god, that could have been me."

I still had one foot in the corporate world of CEOs, and I didn't always feel like I fit in with the yoga crowd. I was still a little put off by some people I met at yoga conferences, who looked like they had wandered out of a time warp from Haight-Ashbury circa 1969 and asked that everyone call them "Moon Spirit." However, the message and power of yoga drew me deeper into the yoga community, where I was experiencing new sensations all the time. The deeper I went into understanding how and where I could serve, the less I spent in the corporate world. But I also felt as though I was in a unique position to build a bridge between those worlds.

As far back as I could remember, I was destined for the corporate world. Although for years it served me well, now that I could reflect back, I realized that going as far back as college I was seeing things differently. I didn't have the courage or strength to do anything about it then, and for several decades I continued down a path that just didn't feel right. I now felt I was making the body and mind connection and starting to live an authentic life, becoming the person I knew existed deep inside of me.

— — —

In addition to looking at my life and choices differently, I was changing my mind about a lot of things. I was never very touchy-feely when it came to prison reform. I thought if someone did the crime, they should do the time, but it is impossible to take a hard look at this country's system of incarceration—which impacts a greater percentage of its populace than any other country on earth—without seeing the desperate need for major changes. As a compassionate person it hurt to see the human cost and from an economic standpoint, as a businessman and accountant, I think every taxpayer should be appalled at the waste and inefficiency in the current system.

Even those who follow a hard line on law and order, who want to lock up the bad guys and throw away the key, should consider that the vast majority of people who are incarcerated will be getting out some day. Is it wise to have them reenter society with no job skills? If they can't get a job, what choice will they have but to turn to the only trade they know? Is it wise for them to reenter society with their anger issues, drug addictions, and mental health problems not only intact but exacerbated by the oppressive and disrespectful environment of prison?

It's hard to see how locking people up for years with no real attempt at rehabilitating them is cost-effective. Most people don't think about prison, but once I had been there, I found it impossible to ignore the massive mess we have on our hands. I know I can't change a giant system, but I have always found it better to light a single candle than to curse the darkness. I can take the healing power of yoga and meditation to those in prison, veterans' centers, and recovery centers. It has been said that often people turn to yoga when they have tried everything else, either for physical healing or emotional healing. I now serve on the boards of other nonprofit groups that are doing their part to change the system or at least make life more tolerable for the people trapped in it.

— — —

For TYP to do its job, we needed instructors to teach the classes, so we began holding training workshops focused on providing tools to serve people dealing with trauma and addiction. Both Colleen and I often share our stories as we develop a safe zone where participants feel safe to open up about their own stories.

At first, I had a hard time admitting I had been in prison. I used to refer to it as "when I was away," never calling it what it was. Now I realized I wasn't being fully honest, and it gave my role in this project more credibility if I told the whole truth. I talk of my former position at a $2 billion company and how instead of bringing me success, it was to be my undoing. I talk about my notion of myself as a "pleaser," but add, "I am still pleasing people, but I am doing it in a positive way." After years of climbing a mountain, the summit of which didn't interest me, I finally found my calling. If my story can somehow help people to cope with their own crisis, I am ready to share.

I also drew on my experience with Bob. For too long I tried to "fix" my brother, and he resented it. When I stopped trying to repair him and just be his friend, things got much better. If we call what we are doing "helping" or "fixing," that implies we are better than the person we are helping. It's better to think of it as serving someone else. How can we serve them? When we want to "cure" people instead of helping them to heal, it leads to co-dependency. We need to give people space and support to find their own ways. This is all part of nondualism and having to stop seeing ourselves as different or apart from others.

I asked those who attended my trainings that what we said in the room stayed in the room. I wanted it to be a safe zone where people felt comfortable opening up. Often, just in sharing their stories people would cry and get others crying. Whether these trainings are held in economically depressed parts of the city or upper-middle-class suburbia, the stories I would hear would often be similar.

At one training, a woman said she practices yoga to cope with the pressure of her daughter's addiction and realized she could help others in a similar situation as well as the addicts who were the source of others' stress. Another participant had been a medic in Iraq, and after his experience he got into yoga to heal his own emotional wounds, now wanting to help others overcome theirs as well. Others spoke of having loved ones in prison and wanting to help them by proxy. One woman said her son had died of a drug overdose, and she wanted to use yoga to help others in recovery so that no one else suffered the same fate. It was hard not to get emotional hearing their motivations.

During one class I taught at a VA hospital, I noticed that one of the men was wearing an ankle bracelet. Then I noticed another. Now that I was looking, I could see everyone in the class but me had the monitoring device. It crossed my mind to wonder why, but I quickly decided it was better if I didn't know. I wasn't there to judge or condemn them, someone had already done that. We teach regardless of who the person is and without an expectation of changing anyone. We simply provide the tools for the participants to become their own teacher. If they are willing to work on themselves, then I should be willing to work with them. And if in bettering themselves, it makes for a better world, then why wouldn't I do my part? I would accept them as what they were in this moment with me in this class: people who were seeking a change, a way to better their lives. It was living in the moment: what they did before didn't matter. What mattered is what they were doing now.

One of the tenets of yoga is to always do your best, without being worried about the outcome. This is especially true when serving underserved populations. In one such class, there was a morbidly obese guy who could barely move, let alone do most of the poses, and I assumed he was having a miserable time, as for three weeks he never said a word. Then one day he stayed after class and told me the experience was life-changing. I never saw him again and, under the rules of doing classes in recovery centers or the VA, I'm not supposed to ask why people are there or for how long. All I can do is send him positive thoughts and hope that I was of some service to him. I'll likely never know.

Many people who do this work say that their students always thank them for the class, but we, the teachers, get so much more from the participants. I blogged about one such case for the TYP website:

Yesterday as I drove to SCI (State Correctional Institution) Graterford prison for Transformation Yoga Project's weekly men's yoga/mindfulness class, I wasn't in the best of moods. My body was incredibly itchy from a bad case of poison ivy. You see, the day before I spent the afternoon weeding in the backyard and wandered into a large patch of the green stuff. Poison ivy and I have had a complicated relationship over the years. Every year I vow to avoid getting anywhere near it but the temptation of a weedless garden seems to pull me into the poisonous patch.

Anyway, at the beginning of each class I ask the men to inwardly check in on 3 levels: physical, emotional, and, if so desired, spiritual. I mentioned that physically, I was a bit off due to the relentless itching from poison ivy. We then proceeded with our normal 75-minute (somewhat vigorous) trauma- informed yoga practice. After class it's customary for us to check back in and address any questions about the practice or yoga in general. It was at this point when an inmate came up and said, "Mr. Mike, I know you are having some discomfort with your rash, but I'd give anything for a little poison ivy, as it would mean that I was outside; truly outside, out of the prison yard." His words hit me hard and it brought flashbacks to my own journey and how we take so much for granted. Getting poison ivy means that I'm free; free to make the decision to weed or not; it means that I'm outside in nature and able to enjoy all that we have. Our gift of yoga is to offer the same possibilities to those who have less freedom. We constantly repeat our mantra that "yoga allows us to find comfort in discomfort" and that the poses are a metaphor for life's discomforts.

I have a new appreciation for poison ivy.

I also had seen firsthand the need for people to understand that yoga was not just what happened on the little stretch of real estate that is the mat. In some places we didn't even have mats. It's amusing to watch people in a yoga studio stake out their territory with their mat and towel and water bottle, marking off their personal space. Stepping on someone else's yoga mat is almost sacrilege, like walking between a golfer and the hole while he is putting. I wanted the people in the program to understand that the biggest part of yoga was what happened off the mat.

Occasionally during my classes, I would test a student's calm by deliberately stepping on his mat. I would see if he fell out of the pose or started tensing up. I would talk to him and the rest of the class about what I was doing and ask him if he could maintain his composure in spite of my clear provocation and violation of his personal space. This was a simple test. But the next time someone cuts in front of you in the chow line, can you handle it as well?

— — —

When TYP first started, often when I contacted a prison or recovery center I was met with resistance. But in the few short years TYP has been operating, there has been a huge shift in how we are welcomed. In fact, instead of my knocking on doors, prisons, recovery centers, and veterans' centers started contacting me.

We have also started yoga classes within the Philadelphia prison system and will be expanding into other prisons within this huge system, encompassing six prisons and holding some ten thousand people. And we are working with both Montgomery County and Delaware County, Pennsylvania, for both their adult and juvenile facilities. The demand is huge, and administrators are seeing the benefit of our programs. Our next challenge is finding enough qualified teachers to operate dozens of classes without burning people out.

But not everyone is accepting, and we still run into problems. At one of the prisons we visit, the guard who checks us in calls us the "stretch-olas," as in the people who do stretching. Sometimes he'd say it in a mocking way, other times I'd think it was a friendly nickname. I try to think the best of people, but then one day when he found some paperwork out of order, he used it as an excuse to say we couldn't have class. We have a set time for the class and every minute he held us up, we were keeping the participants waiting and losing valuable time with them. I think the guard thought we'd just leave, but knowing how important this was to men who had been the victims of too many broken promises, I wanted to solve the problem and have class. We had been coming for months. If the paperwork hadn't landed on his desk for today's class, who did we have to call to get it? This is the lack of compassion I saw far too often in Lewisburg. But I had to breathe and calmly ask him to make a call.

James Fox said that in the years he has been working his Prison Yoga Project, the change has been massive. Fourteen years ago, when he arrived to teach a class dressed in his yoga clothes, prisoners and guards alike mocked him, often calling him a *faggot*. He had two brave men show up for his first class. PYP has evidence that recidivism is over 20 percent lower after inmates have been part of a yoga program. Now the administration welcomes him, provides support, and has even asked him to create classes for correctional officers. At some prisons where he works, they have now relaxed the thoroughness of the search each time he enters, but at others, even after a decade they still insist he go through a full screening.

James's work is the subject of a study by the University of San Francisco, and I am proud and pleased that USF will also be tracking some of our TYP classes to see what sort of an impact we are having. We want to add to the growing research showing that yoga and other beneficial programs can reduce recidivism. Yoga's benefits in combating addiction and PTSD have also been shown, and we are hopeful that as more evidence is presented, government officials will see the value in funding programs; pennies spent on yoga will save dollars in treatment costs—and I can say that as a former accountant, not as a yogi.

— — —

Things started moving very quickly. I started getting calls from other prisons and recovery centers and even schools. Could we teach classes for them? One of the officials at the Pennsylvania state prison where we teach near Philadelphia told his counterpart at a prison near Pittsburgh about the program, and I was contacted about expanding there. James Fox also had requests from both inside prison and out, asking if there was a program in Western Pennsylvania. We are getting requests from the greater Philadelphia area—into Delaware and New Jersey. In New Jersey there is a prison that specializes in recovery—a full-prison version of the drug program at Lewisburg, which sounds like the perfect place for TYP's programs.

I don't delude myself that James and other dedicated individuals, such as the people at Liberation Prison Yoga in New York, or my group at TYP, are going to reform our prison system. But we can each do what we can. There is the story of a child walking along a beach where thousands of starfish have washed ashore, stranded by the high tide. He is picking up each starfish and putting it back in the water. An old man says to the child, "There are too many starfish. You can't make any real difference." And the child places another starfish back in the water, looks up at the man and replies, "I made a difference for that one."

We won't save them all. I know that. But the letters and thank-yous from those I have served while in the FDC, while in Lewisburg and since I've been out, indicate that we are helping to change lives. We don't control the destiny of our students, and for the vast majority of them we will never know if we have made a difference. But that's not the objective. Our mission is simply to provide practical tools to help those in need to better deal with the stressors in their lives. Some will choose to use these tools and others won't, but our effort is the same regardless of their decisions. We tell our trainees that you can't hold yourself responsible for outcomes. In Don Ruiz's *The Four Agreements*, the fourth agreement is "always do your best." If you have done that as a teacher, you'll have no regrets when you leave. What the students take from the class is ultimately up to them.

Although we still need a lot more financial support, I have found it gratifying that we are getting donations of all sorts of things necessary to expand our work. Some yoga studios have donated space for our trainings. People have donated clerical work. Manufacturers and distributors of yoga mats have donated boxes of them.

— — —

My friends at Lewisburg report that the classes I had started there are still going on, passed down to a few teachers after me. New ones would come in, train their replacements, and then leave themselves. I was also gratified to hear that they still spoke fondly of "Yogi Mike."

It was also heartening to learn that when some new administrators arrived in Lewisburg, over a year after my departure, these new people understood the importance of yoga and meditation and the men's discussion groups and wanted them to succeed. Instead of the noisy gym or begging for time in the chapel, these classes and groups were now allowed to use a better, quieter space. The drug-rehab unit had been off-limits to inmates from the rest of camp, but now they were allowed to sign up and get permission to go to that building for these sessions.

It was gratifying to know that a pebble I had cast into the pond was still sending out ripples years later. Often, when I wondered if I had made the right move, giving up a large salary to work harder than I ever had, to not only not make money, but actually be spending money on this project, I would get a call or a letter from one of the guys telling me what a good influence I had been and a stabilizing force for them at a time when they felt their lives were unraveling. Those messages would make me push on, knowing that TYP was the right path and I, with the help of the many dedicated yogis flocking to the cause, could help many others through it.

One of the rules that haunts ex-cons is that felons are never allowed to visit other prisoners. I guess on some level it makes sense—they don't want people planning crimes. But what the "system" fails to grasp is that often the best support group for former inmates can be each other. AA works for so many people because it's other addicts who have been there, done that, counseling each other, not some outsider lecturing them on the failings of their lives. Who better understands the challenges of reentering society from prison than other guys who have done it?

My crime was a misdemeanor, so there were no restrictions on whom I could see once my probation was over.

Bull and I have gotten together several times since he left Lewisburg. His presence in my life reminds me of a time in Lewisburg that I would never want to revisit, but at the same time I never want to forget. I learned lessons I could never have learned if left wallowing through life as I had known it. Seeing Bull also reinforces that with yoga and guidance, people can change. If I ever doubt why I am working harder than I ever had to make less money than I have in decades, I can talk to Bull and see what a difference this vocation can make. We can push each other toward the goals we set for ourselves.

Our dedicated volunteers have earned the respect of organizations within both the reentry and recovery fields, such that TYP was asked to develop joint programming with them. We share the common mission of having individuals return into our communities and lead a healthy and productive life through yoga, nonviolent communication, and other reentry programs.

Epilogue:
From Penn to Pen to Zen

Where you are doesn't define who you are.
The journey is as important as the destination.

I got a call from another nonprofit that also served the prison population, asking if I would like to join them for the yoga portion of their nonviolent communication retreat inside a local prison. I was familiar with Heart-to-Heart and the good work they did teaching coping skills in prisons, and was eager to say yes. Until I heard where they wanted me to go for these yoga classes: the Philadelphia FDC.

I told them I would get back to them. I dreaded the thought of returning to a place that had caused me so much anguish.

The call had clearly disturbed me. Beverly asked what it was about. I told her.

"Do you want to go?" she asked.

I started to say no, but I did want to go. I wanted to work with Heart-to-Heart. I wanted this chance to expand TYP. But I didn't want to set foot in the FDC ever again. While I hesitated answering, Beverly said, "You told me about the park you stared at from your cell. Do you want to go? We can go, sit on that bench, see how you feel being that close to the building."

The park had become a minor fixation of mine as I studied it from my cell window. I could open up to her about things including my odd pining for that park because with her there was no need to pretend to be the old Mike. The Mike who was always in charge, always in control. She never knew him. She only knew the new me, whomever he was turning out to be.

I had not wanted to see the FDC since I'd left it. In fact, in the months since I had been out, I had been to only Philadelphia once, to see a Phillies game with my brother and niece. The stadium was nowhere near the part of the city where the FDC was located, so there was no chance of seeing it. While I was in the FDC, I swore I would never come to that other part of the city again. I had softened a bit on my vow of "never again," but still I was not eager to see the place that held so many bad memories for me.

Would it help to see the building and visit the park that in some odd little way had come to represent freedom for me? "Think about it," she said. "If you want, we can go this weekend."

Knowing she'd be there for support, that Saturday Beverly and I drove into the city. Until we got there, I had no idea the park was named Franklin Square. The day was chilly, but there were people with their children waiting to ride the small merry-go-round.

I quickly identified the bench that had been the object of my interest from my cell window. I felt a rush of emotions when I sat on it. I counted the floors of the FDC and windows from the edge of the building to figure out which cell had been mine. I wondered if someone in my old bunk was looking down at the park, wishing he was in my place, as I had wanted to trade places with so many visitors to the park. I had looked down and dreamed of such freedom—something beyond a dream—a desire I had never felt before.

I studied the area. There was the Philadelphia police headquarters, the African American Museum, and the local PBS building. I knew if we walked a few blocks over we'd get a good view of the birthplace of America. But my eyes kept coming back to the window that had been mine. The floor above mine was the SHU, the floor below was where Dwayne's associates took his phone calls. Were he or any of his colleagues still in there awaiting trial? I sat for a long time and studied it all. I felt so many things. Relief and redemption. Pangs of sorrow for those still inside who must be longing for this taste of freedom as I did.

I knew I never wanted to set foot in the Federal Detention Center again. It might be too much to say I had nightmares about it, but aspects of it haunted me. For anyone who has never been in such a place, it is hard to paint an accurate picture of it. I am convinced that it's impossible to give anything close to a satisfactory portrayal of what it was like emotionally. The anxiety and pent-up emotions were causing momentary flashbacks, triggering memories and the same traumatic issues I saw in the people I was trying to help. But that was it. I was trying to help! These people needed my help! And what was my own discomfort compared to their suffering? My anxiety would last hours. Theirs would last weeks or months or years. How could I say no?

Heart-to-Heart set up the visit through Dave McCuskey, FDC Philadelphia's Reentry Affairs Coordinator. It was very hard to not take an intense dislike to many of the guards and administrators I encountered along the way for the many reasons I have delineated, from sadism to petty tyranny to incompetence to indifference. None of those qualities were present in Dave McCuskey. He is a compassionate, caring person who is trying very hard to preserve his humanity and that of the people in his care under daunting circumstances. His goal is to return people to the streets in the best possible shape they can be— not an easy task when many of the inmates won't listen or tend to their own betterment, on top of their addiction and mental health issues.

As I thought about my return to the FDC, I was looking forward to meeting Dave. I was looking forward to working with Heart-to-Heart and learning more about their programs. What I was not looking forward to was actually setting foot in a building that had caused me so much grief.

The building looked so different from the outside. As I approached, I could feel my blood pressure rise and my heart begin to race. Why was I so frightened? This visit surely would be different from the last time I was here. For one thing, I could leave at any time. But the place held such anxiety for me that it was hard to disassociate that prior experience with where I was in my life now. I walked past the Dunkin' Donuts where I'd had my last real cup of coffee before I went to my sentencing and then on to prison.

I had never seen the front entrance to the FDC. My previous entry had been through an underground tunnel from the courthouse, and then I'd left at night from the underground bus depot. There was a very small sign indicating this was a prison. I could see my companions from Heart-to-Heart waiting for me. Now I would be going in the front door.

Already it felt less oppressive. In the lobby we identified ourselves to the guard, who was seated behind the bulletproof glass. He called upstairs and we were soon joined by Dave.

I went through the metal detector, signed in, and Dave accompanied us upstairs. There was something liberating about finally being able to ride the elevator like a human being, instead of as a prisoner. I could face the front and watch the numbers flicker on and off. When we got to the floor, it looked exactly the same as the one I had been on, but also completely different. The FDC hadn't changed, but I had. We were shown into the cinder block room, where about ten women waited for us and the class. The woman from Heart-to-Heart asked me to say a few words to them.

I said something that I have repeated in many classes before and since: "Don't let this define your life. This is just a stop on your journey, but not the final one unless you let it be." With the right attitude and perspective, adversity can evolve into wisdom. All of life's events make us who we are, and we are not defined by any one action. I can clearly see that this entire experience was needed to get me to this exact point. I'm right where I should be.

My first trip to the FDC made me a stronger person. It made me a better person. It taught me so much about my inner being, about what is truly important. It taught me who my friends really were. I wish there were a way for everyone to learn the lessons in humility and priorities and service that I gained, without having to go to prison. Now in this return visit, the FDC was showing me that I was indeed on the right path.

I lost so much in going to prison—my reputation, my position, but I found something so much more powerful: a purpose in life. This was to bring yoga to people in need, whether because of incarceration (past or present), addiction, or the stress of war.

I mentioned the idea for this book to a woman—a stranger, really—who said that perhaps this story could help people find a positive outlook for themselves when they, like me, had everything taken away, including their pride (which I learned is far more precious than money) and sense of self.

And what is more important in life than finding a sense of peace and purpose? I now have both.

Joy. Surrender. True self.

Postscript

Beverly and I married in 2016, and she continues to inspire and bring out the best in me. She is actively involved in several nonprofits, including Transformation Yoga Project. We continue to feel blessed that the universe brought us together.

Colleen and I remain close friends. She has taken on a large role at Transformation Yoga Project as an advisor and teacher. She continues to be my teacher and I faithfully attend her 6 a.m. yoga class every Wednesday. Most gratifying is that we now teach together at a maximum- security state prison.

Bull was released in late 2014 and returned to southern New Jersey to start a construction company. He and his wife are working through marital issues as she struggles to forgive him for the impact his actions had on their family. He reunited with his father, who previously disowned him, and now manages his father's business and has an excellent relationship with his children and grandsons. We keep in touch and see each other periodically. He maintains an active meditation and mindfulness practice.

My ex-wife, Jenny, moved to the Jersey Shore where she continues to live. She volunteers for several nonprofits supporting the arts as well as animal shelters, and she has a solid support network of friends. We see each other infrequently, but I am grateful that she attended my father's funeral. We have established a good relationship and periodically talk about issues facing our children.

My oldest daughter, Erin, left her job in Virginia to move to New Orleans to obtain her master's degree. She currently works as a social worker in the sheriff's department in New Orleans. We actively discuss social issues and reform within the criminal justice system.

Upon my release, my youngest daughter, Maria, and I struggled with our relationship. We've worked to improve it and are now in a very good place. She lives outside of Philadelphia and after completing massage therapy school, she currently works at a local fitness center. We get together for breakfast once a month.

Rain Man became chemically dependent while at Lewisburg. Ironically, this prison-induced addiction qualified him for the drug treatment program, allowing him to be released nine months early. He returned to his home in South Carolina, where he got his funeral home license and now works at a funeral home. Toward the end of my time at Lewisburg, he started getting visits from a female from South Carolina who made the long trip to Pennsylvania. They are now married.

Sarge remains in Lewisburg. The appeal that he spent so much time working on was ultimately denied, and he has a few more years to serve. As far as I can determine, he still works in the prison kitchen.

After his release, Smitty returned to New York and fought for custody of the four foster kids he and his wife took in prior to his sentencing. They finally adopted the children, increasing his family to nine children. The family moved to Florida, where he works for a property maintenance company.

Steve returned to Buffalo and was able to keep his home, which was in the process of being foreclosed while he was in prison. His daughter now lives with him. He is active in helping returning citizens with career development and speaks publically on this subject.

Moe was released after serving his eight-year sentence, and he returned to Maine to be with his wife and family. He is seventy-three years old. He continued voluntarily to tutor GED students in his free time for his entire sentence.

About the Author
and Transformation Yoga Project

Michael D. Huggins is the Founder and Executive Director of the Transformation Yoga Project. After receiving an undergraduate degree from Villanova University and an MBA from Wharton, he worked his way up to being the Chief Operating Officer, President, and Chief Executive Officer of several medical device firms.

In 2009, Mike pleaded guilty to a misdemeanor along with his employer and three other executives, which landed him in prison for nine months. The high-profile case drew national media attention, and Mike's world unraveled in the blink of an eye as he was whisked to the Federal Detention Center in Philadelphia.

The yoga he had practiced and taught some years before incarceration turned out to be his salvation on the inside.

He declined lucrative offers to return to the corporate world upon his release, and instead founded the non-profit organization: Transformation Yoga Project, which teaches trauma-informed yoga to prisoners, veterans, and those struggling with addiction. Specially trained in applying yoga practices for addiction recovery and trauma-related issues, he remains active in teaching yoga in prisons, as seen in the Huffington Post, CBS, FOX, and NBC News affiliates. He is a frequent speaker on tools for self-empowerment, and the power of yoga as a tool for rediscovering your true self. He is also a contributor to several books that focus on best practices for teaching trauma-informed yoga and mindfulness to under-served populations.

Transformation Yoga Project operates in prisons, drug rehabilitation centers, and veteran support facilities. We also teach yoga for recovery classes at various universities.

For more information please visit TransformationYogaProject.org

Find us on Twitter at @YogaHeals or follow us on Facebook at facebook.com/TransformationYogaProject

Transformation Yoga Project
P.O. Box 762, Kennett Square, PA 19348

Acknowledgements

It would take another book to express the myriad of reasons for my extreme gratitude to Colleen, who introduced me to yoga, guided my path at so many forks, and went above and beyond the call of friendship during my incarceration by being my conduit to the outside world. She put me in touch with James Fox and so many others in the yoga world who would become my mentors, guides, and friends. She, along with Larry and Sharon, made the drive to Lewisburg on almost every visitors' weekend, often driving through the mountains of Pennsylvania in weather that would frighten a dogsled team.

My daughters provided me with a reason to stay strong. To never lose faith in what was right, to give me a light (and a cup of coffee) at the end of a horribly dark tunnel.

My brother Larry and his wife, Sharon, who were with me every step of the way and who provided connection, friendship, and love when it was needed the most.

My siblings Mary and Brendan who, along with their spouses and kids provided a great source of inspiration and strength. Their visits, cards, and books were a true lifeline and a reminder of just how blessed I am to have such a loving and supportive family.

My ex-wife, Jenny, was there for me throughout purgatory and was willing to stick with me through better or worse—and the times in the FDC and Lewisburg were definitely worse. I am grateful that she was willing to visit and, like Larry and Colleen, relay messages to the outside world, and to manage my affairs and deal with a host of problems that she never dreamed would come her way when she said "I do" twenty-eight years earlier.

My friend Viktor, who stood by me in the corporate world and who was my biggest supporter during the transition to yogi. He always came with a pocket full of change to feed the vending machines, which in turn fed me!

My friends who also wrote to me, visited me, and provided me with the sheer comfort of knowing they were there for me, even on those many sleepless and worry-filled nights, are invaluable.

And my new bride, Beverly, who has already taught me so much and whom I appreciate in so many ways as we take these next steps on our paths, side by side.

Finally, I'd like to acknowledge the invaluable insight from Walter Meyer, who provided much-needed structure, direction, support, and compassion in assisting me to document what was up to now stuck inside of me.

Thank You

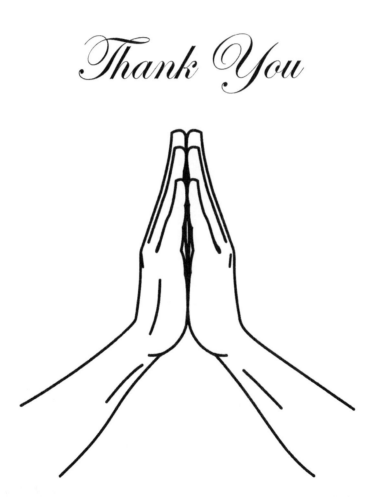

CPSIA information can be obtained
at www.ICGtesting.com
Printed in the USA
BVOW11s0539281116
468990BV00002B/6/P